Successful R Therapy

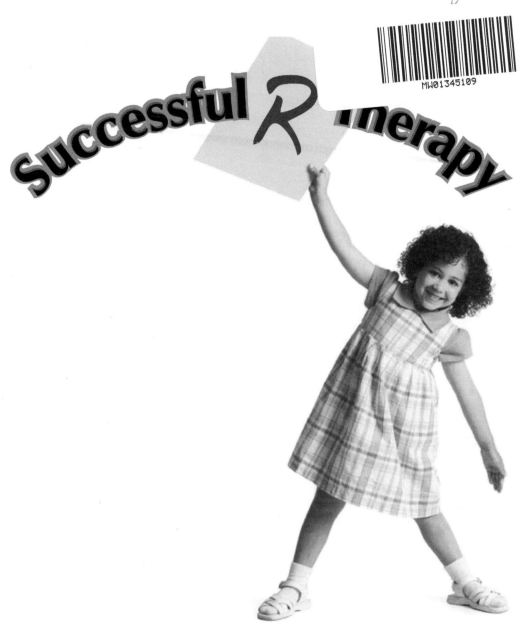

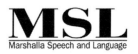

Successful R Therapy
© 2005, 2004 by Pam Marshalla. All rights reserved

ISBN 0-9707060-7-3

Marshalla Speech and Language
11417 - 124th Ave. NE, Suite 202, Kirkland, WA 98033
425-828-4361   Fax 425-828-9891
www.pammarshalla.com

All definitions of speech terms presented in quotes are from *Terminology of Speech Disorders* by L. Nicolosi, E. Harryman and J. Kresheck (Williams and Wilkins: Baltimore. 1983).

The contents of this book may not be reproduced or transmitted in any form or by any means, electronic or mechanical, including photocopying and recording, or by any information storage and retrieval system, without written permission from the author.

Disclaimer
This text describes invasive oral-motor stimulation techniques intended for use by the professional speech and language pathologist. The book has been written with the knowledge that some readers are new to the area of oral-motor therapy while others are well-versed in it. Professionals who utilize these techniques must have thorough knowledge of the oral mechanism, including its structure, sensitivities, reflexes and movements. Professional judgment and common sense must rule the application of these techniques with specific clients. As such, the reader is solely responsible for discretionary use of the oral-motor techniques contained herein.

Dedication

To Dr. Robert K. Simpson, who modeled a deep respect for traditional articulation therapy, and to Ruth Ann who hungered to understand it.

To Alex and Robert, who worked so hard to conquer their R sounds; and to Sharon and Nancy, who supported their boys' efforts so well.

Please Note

- Male pronouns (*he, him, his*) will be used throughout the text to refer to clients.
- Female pronouns (*she, her, hers*) will be used to refer to speech and language pathologists, teachers and other adult helpers.
- The term *normal* will be used to indicate the absence of speech impairment, as in the sentence, "The W-for-R substitution is expected in normal speech development."
- The terms *speech and language pathologist, speech pathologist, speech therapist, speech trainer, speech teacher, facilitator* and *therapist* will be used interchangeably throughout the text.
- All cases described in the text have been taken from the author's direct clinical experiences. Names have been changed to protect privacy, except where clients have asked that their real names be used.

Symbols Used in the Text

Professional speech and language pathologists use the International Phonetic Alphabet (IPA) to transcribe the spoken word. This is a good thing because it allows a report writer to specify exactly how a client is speaking specific phonemes. Such precision means, however, that there are at least ten different phonetic symbols used to signal differences in stress and pronunciation of the phoneme that is the subject of this book. Such a great number of symbols makes writing even the simplest sentence extremely cumbersome. The title of this book, for example, would read: *Successful /ɚ/, /ɝ/, /aɚ/, /iɚ/, /uɚ/, /oɚ/, /eiɚ/, /aiɚ/, /auɚ/, and /ɔiɚ/ Therapy.* Yikes!

In order to simplify this material, it became necessary to develop a symbol that could represent all forms of our subject sound. Toward this end, the following procedures have been adopted:

- The capital letter R has been chosen to stand for our subject phoneme in all its variations. This nonstandard simple designation allows us to discuss the production of /ɚ/, /ɝ/, /aɚ/, /iɚ/, /uɚ/, /oɚ/, /eiɚ/, /aiɚ/, /auɚ/, and /ɔiɚ/ as a collective whole. It also makes the text more readable by the concerned public.

- Isolated capital letters also have been used throughout the text to designate all other consonant phonemes. For example, L is used for /l/. Uppercase letters also are used for the vowels. For example, E is used for /i/.
- A combination of upper and lowercase letters is used to designate phonetic symbols that require the use of two or more standard orthographic symbols and blends. For example, Sh is used for /ʃ/, Ng is used for /ŋ/, Br is used for /br/ and Spr is used for /spr/. Some vowel sounds also are designated with a combination of upper and lowercase letters. For example, Ah is used for /ɑ/.
- Standard orthographic spellings are used where nonsense words have been employed to explain procedures. For example, *bar-bar-bar* is used for /bɑɚ bɑɚ bɑɚ/.
- Where it has been necessary to use IPA symbols, Standard English spellings appear alongside.

Contents

Introduction   9

1. The Incredible R   13
   Basic Facts about a Most Difficult Phoneme

2. Understanding the Problem   29
   The Misarticulations of R

3. Assessing the Details   45
   A Deep View of R Misarticulation

4. Achieving the Impossible   59
   Real Work with Real People

5. Listening and Learning   75
   The Essential Work of Auditory Stimulation

6. Seeing It Clearly   91
   Visual Input Makes the Work Concrete

7. Positioning the Tongue for a Tip R   101
   Methods to Teach the Grand Sweep

8. Positioning the Tongue for a Back R   117
   How to Attain a Nearly Impossible Position

9. Locking in on the Cornerstone R   129
   Assure Success with a Solid Foundation

10. Building the Transition Repertoire   141
    Word Inventories of Careful Construction

11. Adapting to New Sensations   177
    Tactile and Proprioceptive Sensation and New Phoneme Acceptance

12. Capturing the Client's Attention   185
    How to Engage, Inspire and Motivate Participation and Carryover

13. Assuring Persistent Success   211
    Final Words of Advice on Successful R Therapy

Glossary   215
References   223
Appendix A: Functional Zones of the Tongue   225
Appendix B: Sample Evaluation Report   227
Appendix C: Sample Letter to Physician   229

Introduction

For more than twenty-five years, I have traveled to all four corners of the United States and Canada teaching continuing education seminars on the longterm persistent R distortion. Speech and language pathologists everywhere struggle with this so-called "mild" articulation disorder because it is not always easy to fix. While many clients learn this sound quickly and easily, great numbers simply cannot pronounce R no matter what. Correct production of the sound becomes the client's unobtainable and elusive Holy Grail, and the R sound they are left with sounds very bad. The speech and language pathologist who is in charge of this client's failed speech program usually feels terrible when this occurs.

Unfortunately, articulation therapy for mild cases has gone out of favor as the primary responsibility of the speech and language pathologist. Throughout the past twenty years, therapists have been required to give less time to clients with mild speech problems and more time to those with severe speech and language disability. Simultaneously, university training programs have deemphasized phonetics and articulation training. As a result, thousands of children with distorted R's are left untreated either because therapy has been taken away from them or because the assigned therapist has not been taught how to fix the problem in the first place. I find this to be a tragedy for bright children with this error. These children are our future leaders in politics, medicine, scientific research, education, religion, mathematics, music, theater, publishing and more. They deserve to have good speech with clarity on all phonemes. As a society, we need them to be able to communicate their ideas clearly.

My greatest interest in the profession of speech and language therapy has always leaned toward the speech side. In university, I loved my classes on the anatomy and physiology of speech movement, and I had the great privilege of studying under Dr. Willard Zemlin, author of the acclaimed *Speech and Hearing Science*. I also excelled in phonetics and phonology under the careful tutelage of Dr. Elaine Pagel Paden and the enthusiastic clinical work of Dr. Barbara Hodson, joint authors of the infamous phonology primer, *Targeting Intelligible Speech*. I also learned articulation development, assessment and therapy in undergraduate courses taught by a relatively unknown yet dedicated professor, Dr. Robert K. Simpson. Dr. Simpson was a proponent of traditional articulation therapy, ala Dr. Charles Van Riper. He taught us the nuts and bolts of treatment, and he had a way of helping us to think about the process of changing speech habits. After graduate school, I was introduced to the development of oral movement in feeding by Dr. Suzanne Evans Morris while she was undertaking a doctorate at Northwestern University. *Voilé!* The concept of oral-motor therapy in articulation and phonological therapy was born. These five teachers have had a huge influence on my work, and their teaching paved the way for all of my written work, including this current volume.

I began to study oral movement as it related to speech sound production, phonetics and phonology. My first public presentation on the topic was a paper on the lateral lisp presented at the Illinois Speech and Hearing Association Convention in 1979. My first two-day workshop on oral-motor therapy was presented in 1982. It was entitled *Tactile and Proprioceptive Stimulation Techniques in Articulation Therapy*. There were fifty people in attendance. Since then, the topic of oral-motor therapy has become a hot topic in the field of speech and language therapy as more therapists have become interested in its methodology. Oral-motor therapy dominated the field during 1990s and has continued its strong presentation into the twenty-first century in the therapy rooms of this country.

A predictable problem in the widespread use of oral-motor techniques has ensued, however. In our profession, we tend to let go of old ideas as we grab hold of new ones. Following this tendency, therapists have begun to substitute oral-motor techniques for traditional articulation therapy procedures. For example, I received a call recently from a speech and language pathologist who was concerned about her client with a lateral lisp on all the sibilants. She assured me that she had read everything I had written on oral-motor therapy, and that she even had attended a few of my seminars on the subject. She said that she "believed" in oral-motor therapy. Then she stated that although she had helped the client improve his basic jaw, lip and tongue control, he still could not produce a midline sibilant. She wondered what else she could do. She wanted more advanced oral-motor techniques. But she did not need any. What her therapy procedures were missing was basic information about the phonemes themselves. She and her client were not working on phonemes; they were working on oral movements. His oral-motor skills were improving, but his phonemes were not.

This is a wrong approach.

One does not engage in oral-motor therapy and then assume that all phonemes will fix themselves simply by practicing them over and over again. Instead, oral-motor techniques should be embedded into an articulation or phonological therapy program that addresses the phonemes or phonological processes in error. Oral movement should be taught side by side with other methods of speech sound awareness and production. This book is a demonstration of that idea. It explains how one integrates oral-motor therapy procedures into a traditional program of articulation therapy for the remediation of R.

I have presented the best I can about articulation therapy for the misarticulated R phoneme in this volume. The perspective arises from a combination of ideas from phonetics, phonology, oral-motor therapy, behavior management, language development, child development, psychology and, of course, my own nearly three decades of clinical experiences. It has not been an easy book to write, and I have gone through numerous drafts over more than twenty years to do it. I have found that it is difficult to translate the dynamics of therapy onto the written page. To describe with words what one hears with the ears, sees with the eyes and feels with the hands has proven to be arduous. And to describe what one feels with the heart and intuits with the mind during the course of treatment is almost impossible. It is much easier to explain all these things in the workshop format during which models can be offered and videotapes can be shown. The visual image fills many gaps left behind by the written word. Throughout this writing I have tried to avoid all standard reporting protocols. I have instead written this book as if you the reader were sitting with me and I was simply describing to you what I know. I have not tried to prove my techniques; I have only tried to explain them.

Currently, I operate a private practice in the Seattle suburbs, and I see preschool and school-age children with a wide variety of speech and language problems. My caseload always contains elementary, junior-high and high-school students with persistent R distortion. I usually see lots of R kids in the summer, and I provide consultation throughout the year to area therapists needing help with these kids. I also tend to serve the offspring of speech and language pathologists. I love the intricacies of R production and its distortion, yet I am ever intimidated by the challenge a new client brings to therapy. With each new case I ask myself, "Can I help this one?" Honestly, I almost always doubt my skill at the onset of treatment. Then the therapy itself reveals to me whether or not I know what I'm doing. Direct treatment always forces me to change and improve my techniques. At this point, some 28 years into my career, I think I am finally ready to write down that which has proven successful for me in R therapy.

Readers will come to this book with various levels of expertise in articulation therapy. If you are a well-seasoned therapist, this material will reinforce what you already know. It will help you understand what you are doing, and it may help explain your plans and procedures to clients, parents and other colleagues. If you are new to the field of speech and language therapy, if you are new to R therapy, or if you are simply struggling with R therapy, you need two things: information and experience. You will get lots of information here, but hands-on experience only comes with time. Skill in treating an R distortion is perfected during years of direct work with a wide variety of clients. Learn what to do here, but pay careful attention to what you are doing in your treatment room. Also, seek hands-on help from other therapists who work in your geographic area. Thirty minutes of watching and talking with another more experienced therapist can reveal secrets of therapy that written material simply cannot.

This is not a cookbook of R therapy techniques. Dr. Simpson, to whom this book is dedicated, would give me fifty lashes with a wet noodle if it were. However, these practical ideas have been presented in such a way that the reader would be helped to *think* about the misarticulation of R. Ultimately, what makes for successful R therapy is the ability to see the issues clearly and to think through the remediation process. I have included exercises throughout the text to help readers learn the basic ideas presented here. These exercises represent the types of successful real-life experiences I have used in my workshops on R therapy. I also have made illustrations to clarify points.

My hope is that the information presented in this book will serve speech and language pathologists and their limitless supply of clients with longterm persistent R misarticulation.

I also hope that this book will help stimulate the field of speech and language therapy to return once more to the scientific study of phonetics and articulation remediation. Seasoned professionals familiar with the works of Dr. Charles Van Riper and his colleagues will be pleased to see so many of the "old ideas" brought back to life. New studies on articulation development, disorder and remediation that are based on current information about oral-motor development could make these research projects fantastic. In fact, there are thousands of statements in this book that could be the cornerstone of any number of research projects. The information discovered in them would further the knowledge that the professional speech and language community needs to improve their worldwide services to clients with R misarticulation.

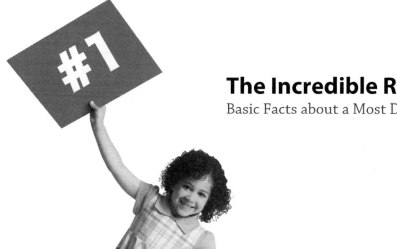

The Incredible R
Basic Facts about a Most Difficult Phoneme

Correct pronunciation of the North American English R is so difficult to master that some English speakers fail to learn it and face a lifetime of whispered ridicule.

- "He talks funny."
- "What's wrong with him?"
- "Is he from somewhere else?"
- "I don't think he's very smart."

Despite the difficulty many people face in attempting to master this sound, the problem of the misarticulated R phoneme is considered a mild one. In fact, many speech and language pathologists do not treat R problems within the public school setting any more. The attitude is that a distorted R does not interfere with a student's academic success. Thus, there is no reason to address it in the academic environment. This attitude about R, and about mild articulation problems in general, also is pervasive in the university training programs that prepare students to become professional speech and language pathologists today. A great number of these advanced degree programs have reduced the amount of time spent on phonetics and articulation so much that new graduates report they have never discussed the distorted R in class nor have they ever seen a patient with the problem. This is a shame because the distorted R is an extremely common articulation error pattern and its presence is not a minor problem for the person afflicted with it.

Failure to acquire the R sound can cause problems for both children and adults. These people can have trouble being understood and being accepted. They can have difficulty with self- expression and public speaking. Even with high intellectual skills, people with R distortion can be viewed as lacking in intelligence and common sense. Elementary children with distorted R's are called "babies" by their peers, and older students are isolated and considered "weird." Further, despite the popular notion that an R distortion does not interfere with academic success, many of these children have difficulty differentiating the sound of R from other phonemes, especially the vowels. This can result in reading, writing and spelling problems and deficits in general vocabulary acquisition.

Despite these potential problems, however, many people with R distortion blaze through life without ever correcting it. In my travels across the United States and Canada, I have encountered R problems in teachers, preachers, accountants, taxi drivers, film directors, writers, police officers, fire fighters, physicians, grocery store clerks, hotel managers, professors and computer software designers, to name just a few. Even politicians, television journalists and actors, people for whom public speaking is a way of life, can have difficulty with R. Clearly an R distortion does not stop one's life; it merely alters it.

In special cases, an R that is pronounced differently than the crowd can be a good thing. Consider the dialectical speech pattern of President John F. Kennedy with his Massachusetts' R sound, or journalist Barbara Walters with her famous distortion of R. These renowned pronunciations of R and other phonemes have helped them stand out from the crowd. Since an R distortion is attention grabbing, sometimes it is created purposefully for special effect. For example, the unique voices of Bugs Bunny, Elmer Fudd and Tweety Bird were created in part by modifying their R sounds. A variation in the pronunciation of R even can enhance the marketability of a child actor because it makes him appear younger and more innocent or adorable—at least for a few sweet years before he reaches adolescence. In short, when a distortion of R is wanted, it can be a beneficial thing. But an unwanted R distortion is not a good thing when the person afflicted with it cannot get rid of it.

The sound of R is so difficult to produce that it is a wonder small children ever learn to say it correctly in the first place. However, millions of children learn it every day without special help. Most of these children learn it during the preschool years, and nearly all have mastered it by five or six years of age. Only a small percentage has not figured it out by six, seven or eight years of age. These are the children who usually are taken to the speech and language pathologist. If the child's R problem is not part of a more serious speech disorder, most of these children will succeed in acquiring the sound of R after a period of therapy. A small portion fails miserably. These children eventually give up or are dismissed from therapy when it is ascertained that R simply is too hard for them to learn. A failure in learning to say R correctly during many years of speech and language therapy can be exhausting and exasperating for the client as well as his therapist and family. Extensive therapy can take away from time in the classroom learning other subjects, and it can be expensive if done in the private sector.

What is it that the client with persistent R distortion cannot achieve? In the rest of this chapter we shall describe phoneme R as it is pronounced correctly in Standard North American English. We shall describe its acoustic quality and its method of production. We shall discuss the Tip R, the Back R, the Vocalic R and the Consonantal R. We shall describe the oral movements necessary to achieve the correct acoustic quality of the R sound, and we shall discuss why our clients have difficulty acquiring this sometimes elusive phoneme.

Methods of assessment and treatment will be described in the remaining chapters, but readers are cautioned against jumping ahead. All assessment and treatment techniques are based on a thorough understanding of the phoneme itself. This understanding comes from an acoustic and an oral-motor perspective. There has been such a neglect of this topic for so many years that it is necessary to review what we know about R from a traditional phonetics perspective, as well as from a newer oral-motor viewpoint. This material lays the foundation for all of our methods of treatment. It explains why successful techniques are designed the way they are.

The R Sound

The acoustic quality of the R phoneme is at the heart of our discussion about R and at the very core of all remediation techniques. The R phoneme is a sound of unusual distinction. It rings with a quality unmatched by any other consonant or vowel. When articulated correctly in words, phrases, sentences, conversational speech or singing, the R sound goes completely unnoticed. If mispronounced, however, it sticks out like a sore thumb.

The R sound is represented orthographically by the letter we write as capital *R* or lowercase *r*, the eighteenth letter of the alphabet. The R sound:

- Can be strong, as in the word *run*
- Can be weak, as in the phrase *cat or dog*
- Can occur at the beginning, middle or end of words
- Can act as a consonant or a vowel
- Can occur in consonant clusters (blends)
- Is classified as a linguapalatal glide in phonetic terms
- Is characterized as both [+vocalic] and [+consonantal] in phonological terms
- Is made upon exhalation and with voice
- Is made with good oral resonance and without nasality

Other consonants that are characterized similarly and that are most like R include the other three glides W, Y and L. Thus, the R sound makes the word *rate* sound different from *wait* or *late*, and makes *ram* sound different from *yam*. The R sound contributes to a speaker's overall intelligibility. When spoken correctly, the R sound does not draw attention to itself or to the speaker.

Auditory Skills

Clients in R therapy have various amounts of knowledge about their R misarticulations. Some are completely unaware that they have this problem. Others have a vague notion that they don't speak well but do not know that R is a concern. Some clients know they cannot say R and want to fix it, while others know of the problem but don't care that it's there. Regardless of a client's particular recognition or acceptance of the problem, the first step of treatment always is to make the situation known to him. This knowing generally comes through *auditory discrimination* activities.

Auditory discrimination is the ability to distinguish between sounds. For the production of R, a client must be able to distinguish R in two ways. First, he must recognize R as unique from all other consonant and vowel sounds. Second, he must differentiate the correct production of R from any distortion thereof. Many long-term R clients cannot tell whether they are producing good sounds or bad ones. It is amazing to observe them when they think they are producing excellent R's. Many of them have no idea how bad they sound!

The case of Brian illustrates this point. Brian came to me at the age of eleven years. His mother informed me ahead of time that he did not want to come to therapy, so we scheduled a one-time visit for a short assessment and a talk. Brian did not produce one single R sound correctly during that hour, but he assured me that he sounded just fine. He told me that nobody noticed anything about his speech, except his mom and his former speech teacher whom he thought was "stupid." When I asked him to produce his very best R, he made a sound with even worse distortion. When asked how he thought he had done on that task, he said, "That was the best R I ever did!"

Many children have not developed a correct auditory category for the sound of R. They can hear R and they are aware of it as a unique sound, usually. But they cannot hear that their own sound is out of the range of acceptability for the R sound. They have blended correct and incorrect productions of R into one gigantic acceptable group. Our job is to help them make two separate categories out of this: one for good productions and another for bad ones. Techniques to facilitate improved auditory discrimination of R are discussed thoroughly in chapter 5. The ability to differentiate correct from incorrect R sounds is at the heart of learning to say R.

But there is an even more important reason to address auditory discrimination skills in R therapy. It is the ear that teaches the mouth to position correctly. That's right: The ear teaches the mouth to move. We want the client to experiment with subtle changes in jaw, lip and tongue position while listening carefully to the way in which his vocal productions alter with each minute change. The client must listen more carefully to these auditory shifts in his speech than he has listened to anything since his infancy. He must come to hear how his oral-position changes alter his own sound, and he must use this combined auditory-oral-motor experience to figure out how to make a correct R. This is the essence of R therapy. As the reader shall see in chapter 5, we begin with gross auditory discrimination of the therapist's production and end with the client's ear finely tuned to his own sound.

Oral-Motor Skills

How does one make an acceptable R? Any phoneme, including R, is made with certain jaw, lip, tongue and velar movements.

- *Jaw:* Jaw position is relatively the same no matter how one produces a good R sound. It is held slightly lowered so that the mouth is partially open. We call this a *finely graded open position*. The finely graded open position is low enough to allow sound to be emitted from the mouth without muffling, and high enough to allow swift and accurate lip and tongue movement for sound production.
- *Velum:* Velar position also is always the same no matter how one produces a good R sound. It is elevated to prevent the sound from entering the nasal passageways. This makes R oral and not nasal.
- *Lips and Tongue:* The lips and tongue can be positioned in two very different ways that have had various names in the articulation literature. We shall call them the *Tip R* and the *Back R*. Each is discussed individually below. The vocabulary used to describe these movements for R is based on the zones of the tongue proposed in *Oral-Motor Techniques in Articulation and Phonological Therapy*. (See appendix A for an introduction.)

The Tip R

The *Tip R* derives its name from the position of the tongue tip. It also has been called the *Tip-Up R*, the *Tip-Back R*, the *Curled R*, the *Retroflex R*, the *Immature R* and the *Incorrect R*. We shall use the term *Tip R* throughout this text.

The Tip R usually is easier to produce than the Back R. To produce the Tip R, the tongue-tip elevates and curls back toward the velum in a grand sweep. As the tip curls back, the sides of the tongue, from the tip all the way to the back on either side, also curl. In essence, the tongue scoops up in a cup—or bowl—shape and tilts toward the back of the mouth. The middle of the tongue remains low relative to the sides and tip. The overall shape the tongue assumes for a Tip R is like a small cave whose open side is facing the oropharynx. Readers familiar with oral-motor development will recognize this position as an exaggerated tongue-bowl position. The rear-facing cave of the Tip R creates a resonance chamber for the sound of R. If we think of the mouth itself as a resonance chamber, then the correct sound of Tip R is achieved with voice resonating into two chambers: a small resonance chamber formed by the tongue inside a larger resonance chamber formed by the mouth. The walls of the inner chamber shaped by the tongue have a certain firm consistency created by a required level of tension in the tongue's musculature. The lips may retract slightly during production of the Tip R to shorten the length of the oral cavity.

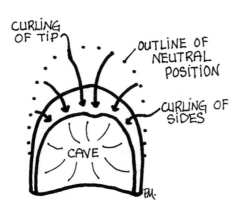

Fig. 1. Aerial View of Tip R Position: Note that both the tip and sides of the tongue are curled up and back to form a small resonance chamber facing the oropharynx.

Fig. 1.1. Lateral View of the Tip R Position: Note that both the tip and sides of the tongue are curled up and back to form a small resonating chamber facing the oropharynx.

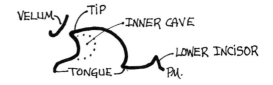

EXERCISE 1.1
Discover Your Habitual R

Discover the type of R you habitually produce. Slowly say the following words aloud: *are, car, bar, jar, star, far* and *bizarre*. Notice the amount of jaw movement and lip rounding you use to achieve R. Then think about your tongue. Does your tongue tip go up and back toward the velum to produce a Tip R? Or does the back of your tongue activate to produce a Back R? What about when you say R at the beginning of a word? Say: *rock, real, room, rich, rack,* and *red*. Do you use a Tip R or a Back R? Do you use both R sounds depending upon word position?

The Back R

The Back R derives its name from the position assumed by the back of the tongue. It has also been called the *High-Back R*, the *Correct R*, the *Mature R* and simply *R*.

In my work with tens of thousands of speech and language pathologists in North America, I have found that most have an incorrect idea about how the tongue actually positions itself for production of the Back R. The standard belief is that the entire back of the tongue elevates toward the velum for production of this sound. This is incorrect. If one were to elevate the entire back of the tongue in one mass toward the velum to produce R, the result would be a sound with distortion.

Rather than functioning as a single unit, the Back R is made through differential control of three parts of the back of the tongue: the middle back and two lateral back sections. In true production of the Back R, the back-lateral margins of the tongue elevate and are braced upward against the molars or palate on either side. They are the points of stability for all tongue movements, including those used in the production of R. With the lateral margins stabilized, the tongue's middle back tenses up toward the velum but does not touch. The tip tends to retract into the body of the tongue as the back sections elevate. Elevation of the tongue's back-lateral margins forms a midline channel for sound to travel through the mouth. Tension of the middle section alters the channel so that R will result. In sum, Back R is made by stabilizing the tongue at its back-lateral margins as the middle back tenses and the lips round.

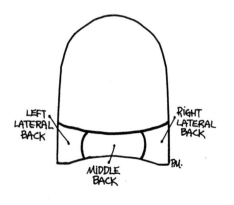

Fig. 1.2. Back of the Tongue: The back of the tongue is comprised of three parts: the middle back and two lateral back sections.

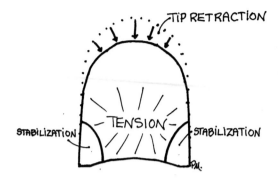

Fig. 1.3. Aerial View of Back R Position: Note that the lateral margins of the tongue are stabilized, the tip is retracted and the middle section tenses.

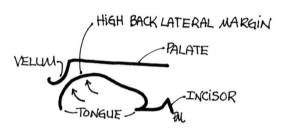

Fig. 1.4. Lateral View of the Back R Position: A true lateral view shows high elevation of the back-lateral margins.

Fig. 1.5. Posterior View of the Back R Position: The posterior view shows that the lateral back sections are stabilized in a high position and that the middle tenses but does not touch the palates.

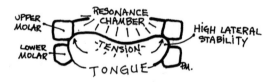

What Is Normal?

Which R is normal, is it the Tip R or the Back R? Most practicing therapists today were taught that the Back R is a superior form of R and that there is something wrong or suspicious about the Tip R. However, early research on R revealed that approximately 60 percent of the normal adult population used the Back R as their habitual R formation, and about 40 percent used the Tip R. My informal workshop questions to thousands of speech and language pathologists nationwide about their own R sounds has confirmed these percentages but revealed that, in addition, a small number use both R's depending upon word position and adjacent vowels. These results reveal that it is normal to produce R either way. It also suggests that therapists should feel free to teach both the Tip R and the Back R to their patients.

What makes the Back R seem more normal, or somehow better, is that the Back R configuration keeps the tongue closer to its neutral position. The *neutral position* is the posture assumed by the tongue when it is not engaged in movement. It has also been called the *resting posture* of the tongue. At rest or in neutral, the tongue lies low in the oral cavity. It fits neatly inside the upper dental arch. The upper surface of the tongue tip tends to articulate with the alveolar ridge, the sides tend to rest gently against the sides of the palate, and the middle and back of the tongue tend to rest low and away from the palate. Production of the Back R keeps the tongue closer to this neutral position than does the Tip R. The Back R is made by lifting and tensing the sides and middle with little displacement of the tip. The Tip R, however, pulls the tip up and far back away from the front of the mouth and toward the velum.

As such, the Back R can be incorporated into conversational speech and blends more easily, and it can be used in speech that is lightening fast. The Tip R, on the other hand, draws the tongue tip far away from its neutral position and into the back of the oral cavity. Its use necessitates a slightly slower rate of speech. It can be said, therefore, that the Back R is a more mature form of R from an oral-motor and speech rate perspective. And perhaps these things do make the Back R better. But not all people speak with the same level of articulatory precision and rate. Some people speak slowly and clumsily, while others speak quickly and with great precision. Both are within the normal range. What brings an R sound into the abnormal range is when it no longer sounds like an R. Whether the sound is made more slowly or more quickly is not an issue of concern in the practice of speech therapy as long as accuracy of sound is maintained.

The Consonantal and Vocalic R Sounds

Classic phonetic literature discriminated between two different kinds of R's: the *consonantal R* and the *vocalic R*.

EXERCISE 1.2
Produce Both R's

Can you produce both the Tip R and the Back R? Try each one while saying "are." Say the word slowly each time. You will feel the tongue tip lift and curl back toward the velum if you are using a Tip R. If you are using a Back R, you will feel activity in the back of your tongue. If you habitually use a Tip R, you may have difficulty producing "are" with a Back R. On the other hand, if you habitually do a Back R, you probably will have no problem using a Tip R on "are." This is because the Tip R is easier. It is made with a bigger movement pattern that requires little refinement. The whole tongue engages in one upward and backward scoop. The Back R requires more differentiation of tongue control in the back. The Back R is difficult to learn if it does not come naturally.

CONSONANTAL R

The consonantal R, phonetically transcribed as /r/, occurs in the initial position of syllables and words. It presents as a consonant and it occurs before vowels. For example, the words *run* and *deride* each contain a consonantal R. The word *run* contains an R in the initial position of the word. The word *deride* contains an R in the middle of the word but in the opening position of its second syllable. The consonantal R also is used in mature consonant clusters. For example, the words *scratch*, *truck* and *drain* each contain a consonantal R. The consonantal R can be made with either the Tip R or the Back R.

VOCALIC R

The vocalic R occurs after a vowel and at the end of syllables and words. It is considered a *vocalic* or vowel-like sound. The words *car* and *argue* each contain a vocalic R. The word *car* contains a vocalic R in the final position of the entire word. The word *argue* contains a vocalic R in the final position of the first syllable of the word. Word-final and syllable-final consonant clusters also utilize vocalic R sounds. For example, the word *cars* contains a vocalic R. The vocalic R can be made with either the Tip R or the Back R. The vocalic R is transcribed as /ɝ/ and /ɚ/. The first is used in stressed syllables; the second in unstressed. However, due to the strong co-articulatory effects of the preceding vowel, the transcription of vocalic R is presented as a single phonetic unit with its preceding vowel. Thus, we have several different transcriptions and many different spellings of the vocalic R as listed below:

IPA symbol	SPELLING	SAMPLE WORD
/ɝ/	er	term
	ir	sir
	ur	hurt
	or	word
	ear	earn
	our	courage
	yr	myrtle
	urr	hurry
	ere	were

IPA symbol	SPELLING	SAMPLE WORD
/ɚ/	er	manner
	or	color
	ur	murmer
	ar	altar
	ir	elixir
	yr	martyr
	ure	figure
	ior	junior

IPA SYMBOL	SPELLING	SAMPLE WORD
/iɚ/	ear	dear
	eer	steer
	ere	here
	er	period
	ier	pier
	eir	weir
	ir	spirit

IPA SYMBOL	SPELLING	SAMPLE WORD
/oɚ/	ore	store
	or	for
	oor	door
	oar	oar
	our	court
	ar	warm
	eor	George

IPA SYMBOL	SPELLING	SAMPLE WORD
/eiɚ/	air	chair
	er	very
	err	merry
	ar	canary
	are	spare
	eir	their
	ere	there

IPA SYMBOL	SPELLING	SAMPLE WORD
/uɚ/	ure	pure
	our	tour

IPA SYMBOL	SPELLING	SAMPLE WORD
/ɑɚ/	ar	car
	ear	heart
	er	sergeant
	uar	guard

IPA SYMBOL	SPELLING	SAMPLE WORD
/ɑiɚ/	ire	fire
	igher	higher
	ir	environment

IPA symbol	spelling	sample word
/ɑuɚ/	our	hour
	ower	power

IPA symbol	spelling	sample word
/ɔiɚ/	oyer	foyer
	awyer	lawyer

Many therapists have been led to believe that the consonantal and vocalic forms of R comprise two different sounds. Some even believe that all the R sounds listed above are different sounds. This is confusing. What we need to understand about these sounds is that the oral movement necessary to achieve the correct acoustic quality or *resonance* of R is the same in each of these forms. What is different is what happens around the pure and essential R sound.

On-Gliding, Off-Gliding and Target Position

The real difference between the consonantal and vocalic forms of R lies in voicing as it occurs during the *on-glide* and *off-glide* movements of R. All phonemes including R are made in three basic sequential stages: an *on-glide*, a *target position* and an *off-glide*.

- *On-glide:* The on-glide is comprised of those movements that are made as the oral mechanism moves into position for the R sound. The tongue can on-glide with Tip R or Back R movements. Voicing while on-gliding into R makes it vocalic.

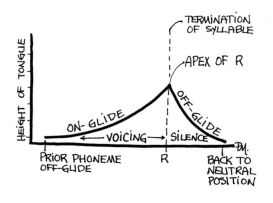

Fig. 1.6. Vocalic R is made by voicing during the on-glide and apex position. Devoicing occurs after the apex.

- *Off-glide:* The off-glide is comprised of those movements that are made as the oral mechanism moves away from the apex of R movement. The tongue off-glides from either the Tip R or Back R target position. Voicing while off-gliding away from R's target position makes it consonantal.

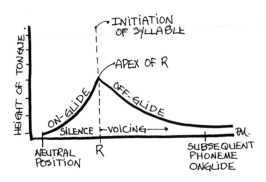

Fig. 1.7. Consonantal R is made by on-gliding in silence. Voice is initiated while the tongue is in the apex position, and it continues during the off-glide.

- *Target Position:* The target position is the apex of speech movement for R. It is the place where the speaker switches from on-gliding to off-gliding. This is where the true acoustic quality or isolated R sound is heard. The isolated R is achieved by on-gliding and off-gliding in silence by voicing during target position. The tongue can employ either a Tip R or Back R position in its target position for the isolated R.

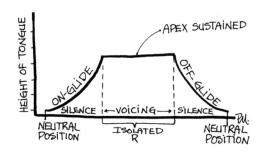

Fig. 1.8. Isolated R is made by on-gliding and off-gliding in silence. Voice is produced only while the apex position is held

EXERCISE 1.3
EXPERIMENT WITH THE VOCALIC R

THE VOCALIC R IS THE SOUND OF R THAT OCCURS DURING THE ON-GLIDE AND TARGET-POSITION PHASES. ITS OFF-GLIDE OCCURS IN SILENCE. SLOWLY SAY *PEER, PAIR, PURR, PORE* AND *PAR* ONE AT A TIME. NOTICE THAT VOICE IS PRODUCED ON THE VOWELS AND CONTINUES AS THE TONGUE GLIDES INTO POSITION FOR EACH R SOUND. NOTICE ALSO THAT VOICING TERMINATES WHILE THE TONGUE IS STILL IN TARGET POSITION FOR EACH R, AND THAT THE OFF-GLIDE IS MADE IN SILENCE.

EXERCISE 1.4
EXPERIMENT WITH THE CONSONANTAL R

THE CONSONANTAL R IS THE SOUND OF R THAT OCCURS DURING THE TARGET POSITION AND OFF-GLIDE PHASES. ITS ON-GLIDE OCCURS IN SILENCE. SLOWLY SAY *READ, RID, RAID, RED, RAD, RUDE, ROOK, ROPE, RAW, ROB* AND *RUT* ONE AT A TIME. NOTICE THAT TARGET POSITION FOR R IS ACHIEVED IN SILENCE, AND THAT VOICE IS INITIATED AFTER THE TONGUE ACHIEVES ITS TARGET POSITION FOR EACH R. ALSO NOTICE THAT VOICE CONTINUES AS THE TONGUE OFF-GLIDES FROM R AND MOVES INTO THE SUBSEQUENT VOWEL.

Why Be Concerned with On-gliding and Off-gliding Features?
It is critical that speech and language pathologists understand how the process of on-gliding and off-gliding impacts the production of the consonantal and vocalic forms of R for two reasons. First, difficult clients treat the vocalic and consonantal forms of R very differently. Any seasoned therapist can report that some clients learn initial-position R, some learn final-position R, others learn R in a certain blend and still others learn a correct R sound but then distort it by adding other sounds to it during the on-glide and off-glide phases. As we shall discuss, these are all on-glide and off-glide problems that need to be thoroughly understood and targeted in therapy.

The second reason that on-gliding and off-gliding is important to understand has to do with the natural acquisition of R by young children. Babies, toddlers and young preschool children do not tend to learn R in isolation. They learn it by experimenting with gliding oral movements produced while prolonging sound. We call this process *babbling*. Babies, toddlers and young children babble with vocalic sounds by prolonging vowels as they move the jaw, lips and tongue into various positions. The sounds of W, L, Y and R as well as all other vocalic speech and non-speech sounds are the result. These sounds are produced haphazardly throughout the babbling process. Children happen upon R while experimenting with sound this way. In fact, they learn all phonemes this way.

Just like the baby or toddler, it can be easier for our clients to learn R while experimenting with oral movements as they prolong vowel sounds. Learning to produce R in isolation by on-gliding and off-gliding in silence is very difficult. In fact, it can be impossible for many a client to understand how in the world he should position the tongue for R unless he has some other sound before or after it to help him understand his movements. The surrounding sounds help him perceive what his tongue is doing. Producing a correct R while simply holding the tongue in either a Tip R or Back R position is challenging, if not impossible, for almost every difficult client. Unfortunately, the traditional methods of articulation therapy proposed that we teach phonemes in isolation first. This is a mistake for many R clients because it ignores the natural process of phoneme learning and the great difficulty one can have in understanding the isolated R position. Therapy to remediate R moves much more quickly when therapists understand the critical role that on-gliding and off-gliding play in treatment. This concept is imbedded throughout the treatment techniques proposed in this text.

— *Summary* —

- Correct production of the Standard English R sound is learned easily by millions of young children who are unaware that they are learning anything special.

- Correct pronunciation of the North American English R is so difficult to master that some English speakers fail to learn it and face a lifetime of whispered ridicule.

- The problem of the misarticulated R phoneme is considered a mild one that often goes untreated. However, an unwanted misarticulation of R can have a negative impact upon the speaker in terms of how others perceive him intellectually and socially and how he perceives himself. Misarticulation of R also can interfere with reading and spelling skills when problems in vowel and glide differentiation are present.

- The acoustic quality of R is very specific and is at the heart of all remediation techniques. Clients with R misarticulation have not made a distinction between the correct acoustic quality of R and their own misarticulation. Our job is to help them make this distinction.

- The oral movements patterns required to produce the Tip R and the Back R are very specific in terms of jaw, lip, tongue and velar position. The primary difference between Tip R and Back R lies in tongue position. The Tip R is made with a grand sweep of the tongue tip as it curls up and back toward the velum. The Back R is made by stabilizing the back-lateral margins of the tongue on the molars or palate while tensing the middle back toward but not touching the palate.

- Both the Tip R and the Back R are normal. Either is an excellent treatment option. Some speakers naturally use both the Tip R and the Back R depending upon phonetic context.

- The Tip R is an easier tongue movement pattern to acquire. It is used by approximately 40 percent of the normal adult population. The Back R is a more difficult oral movement to perceive, even by speakers who have already acquired the sound. However, it is used by approximately 60 percent of the normal adult population.

- The consonantal and vocalic productions of R are essentially the same sound. They are different by voice onset and termination.

- The consonantal R is the sound of R as it occurs at the beginning of a syllable. It is consonant-like. The consonantal R is written with only one IPA symbol: /r/. It is made with either a Tip R or a Back R.

- The vocalic R is the sound of R as it occurs at the end of a syllable after a vowel. It is vowel-like. The vocalic R is written with many different IPA symbols that depend upon the preceding vowel. Vocalic R is made with either a Tip R or a Back R.

- All phonemes are made with a sequence of three basic movements: the on-glide movements, the target position and the off-glide movements. The difference between the consonantal and vocalic R sounds lies in where voicing and devoicing occurs in this sequence. Isolated R is made while the tongue is held in its target position.

- Clients treat the consonantal R and the vocalic R sounds differently because of their on-glide and off-glide properties. An inability to learn both the consonantal and vocalic forms of R often is at the heart of the long-term persistent R misarticulation.

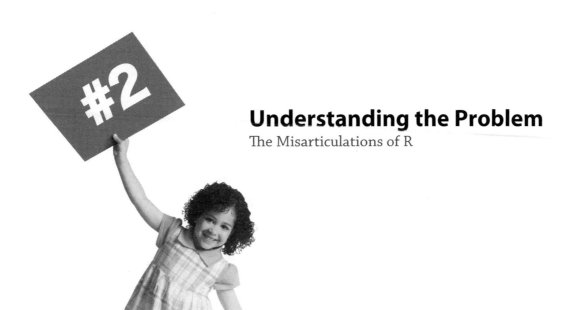

#2 Understanding the Problem
The Misarticulations of R

Now that we understand how to make a correct R sound, we can begin to discuss its misarticulations. We shall describe these from a phonetic perspective and from an oral-motor one. Misarticulation of the R sound occurs in the same basic three ways that any phoneme is altered when affected by speech impairment. That is, by *omission, substitution,* or *distortion*. The following sections discuss common characteristics of these three error types and their occurrence in normal development. Introductory comments about the treatment approach for each are offered here. Particular attention is given regarding the R sound that is affected by distortion because that error is the most problematic and resistant to treatment.

Omission: A Lack of R
When a phoneme is omitted, it is left out altogether. When omission of R occurs, the client might say "ain" for *rain*, "ca" for *car* or "bown" for *brown*. Complete omission of R is observed in young children who have not acquired the sound yet. It also is common in older children with apraxia, dysarthria, severe articulation disorder and phonological delay. Complete omission of R is uncommon, however, when R is the client's only error phoneme.

A complete omission of R is fairly easy to remediate because the client only has to learn new movement. He has no incorrect movements to unlearn. However, in today's practice it is common to ignore a complete omission of R when speech is severely impaired. This is because the client usually has much more pressing and earlier developing phonemes to learn. I disagree with this approach. A better plan is to teach the client to substitute another sound for it. The substitute sound becomes a placeholder for R, a sound from which true R can later emerge.

Substitution: A Replacement for R
More common than the complete omission of R is its substitution. As the name suggests, a substitution occurs when one phoneme is used in place of another. The substitution of another phoneme for R is seen in normal speech development and in severe articulation disorder, as well as in cases of isolated R misarticulation. Consonants that are substituted

for the R consonant most commonly include the other glides—W, L and Y. Of these three, W is the most common in both normal development and in articulation disorder. However, other more unusual substitutions are observed in cases of severe articulation and phonological disorder. For example, D or Ng might be substituted for R.

The typical W-for-R substitution is so common in childhood development that it is viewed as a normal occurrence in early-developing speech patterns and it is classified as a *developmental error*. For example, when saying "I rode a red bike," a typical three-year-old child might say, "I wode a wed bike." People sometimes call this baby talk because it is the way very young children typically speak. In the speech and language literature, the term *labialization* is used for this error. Labialization refers to the substitute of a *labial* (lip) sound for a *lingual* (tongue) sound. A W-for-R substitution occurs because children have not learned the tongue movements necessary for R. They use similar lip movements instead. The W sound makes a good substitute for R for three reasons: (1) it is acoustically similar to R, (2) it is very easy to see, and (3) it can be made with very gross oral movements. The W-for-R substitution is a stop along the path of normal development. Most children are expected to make this stop. However, they should not stay there forever.

The W-for-R substitution that occurs in normal development is outgrown in most cases. If not, a short period of treatment may be necessary. The child with an isolated W-for-R substitution should be able to learn the correct tongue movement patterns necessary for R to emerge quickly and without much difficulty. Even without treatment, many children with a W-for-R substitution acquire R all by themselves during kindergarten or first grade. These children spend considerable time learning all the letters of the alphabet. Good teachers teach the sound each letter makes, and they help their students compare and contrast sounds so that they can discriminate them with greater skill. The child who has not been able to mature past the developmental W-for-R substitution by the end of kindergarten or first grade should receive treatment to help him get past it. It should be noted that this is current practice in many public schools. However, some school systems wait until these children are eight or nine years of age, and others do not treat R at all when it occurs in isolation.

Unlike the W-for-R substitution that is seen in normal development, the W-for-R substitution that occurs with severe speech, language or cognitive disorder may not be outgrown. Clients with severe speech and language disorder often fail to learn a variety of phonemes, including R even after years of treatment. Often it is necessary to allow these clients to continue their W-for-R substitutions into and throughout adulthood. If a severely speech-impaired client uses an uncommon sound as a substitute for R, it is best to train him to use the more common W-for-R substitution instead. This change improves his intelligibility considerably and ensures that more listeners will understand him. It also puts his error on the normal developmental path and allows for the possibility that he eventually will learn a true R.

Distortion: An R Poorly Made

While an omission is a lack of R, and a substitutions a replacement for R, a distortion is the result of bending or contorting the sound. The client with a distortion is in fact attempting to say R, but he fails to achieve a correct acoustic quality because he cannot achieve the necessary on-glide, off-glide or target position for either the Tip R or the Back R. The client has been forced to rely on those movements he can do and those positions he can achieve instead of the correct ones. The client with an R distortion misshapes his mouth for the production of R and is unable to achieve the acoustic result he needs. A distortion of R is by far the most difficult pattern to change because the movement and auditory changes are quite subtle.

A distortion of R is not a developmental error, and it should not be treated as such. It is not a stop along the path of normal speech acquisition. It is an aberration, the result of employing an incorrect oral-movement pattern. To make a distorted R, a child veers off the normal developmental path onto a different one that takes his speech sound in the wrong direction. As such, he can never reach speech maturity because he is heading away from a normal R production. The distorted R is best treated as soon as possible in order to help the client return back to the normal developmental path. This can be done in many cases by teaching the client to make the classic W-for-R substitution. That simple change puts him back on track. From there, a correct R may emerge. If not, very specific treatment must ensue.

It is more difficult to alter an R distortion than it is to change an omission or substitution, because the child must do two things: He must relinquish an old movement pattern and learn a new one simultaneously. Treatment consists of inhibiting the habitual abnormal oral-movement pattern while facilitating a correct and eventually more advanced one. The distorted R pattern is not a minor error pattern, and therapy to correct it can be long term. The process can fail miserably if the client's aberrant oral-motor patterns are ignored or misunderstood. When good oral-motor techniques are included in treatment, however, therapy time can be reduced considerably—from years to months in most cases.

It is tempting to limit our discussion of R therapy in this book to those clients with an isolated R problem. However, the distortion of R occurs in a wide variety of clients, from those with a single phoneme error to those with severe articulation disorder. It is important that we discuss this complete range of possible errors. For the purposes of our discussion, clients with R distortion are organized into three basic categories: those with severe dysarthria, those with mild and perhaps unrecognized dysarthria and those with completely intact oral-motor skill.

Category 1: Distortion with Severe Dysarthria

Distortion of R can be due to a severe motor dysfunction and related oral-motor deficit. For example, the child with cerebral palsy typically has distortion of many sounds including R. Clients with generalized neuromuscular disorder have problems in all movements, including the movements of respiration, phonation, resonation, speech articulation, eating and swallowing. Their characteristic R distortion is the result of differences in muscular development, coordination, tone, oral-tactile sensitivity and basic awareness of oral movement. Dysarthria is the term we use to label speech that is distorted in this way. Thus, R is distorted just like most other phonemes when dysarthria is present.

When an R distortion occurs as a part of a severe neuromuscular disorder, the error is considered only one small part of the client's overall dysarthric pattern. Speech training should focus on general pronunciation and the prosodic elements of speech, including rate, intonation, volume, stress, and fluency. Treatment also should address overall oral-motor control for both speech and feeding. General pronunciation and specific phonemes should be targeted, yet activities designed specifically for R may or may not be included. Inclusion of R into treatment depends upon severity of dysarthria, general goals of treatment and expectations of progress during the period of treatment. The W-for-R substitution may be taught as a placeholder for the correct R that may or may not emerge later.

Category 2: Distortion with Mild Dysarthria

The second category of clients with R distortion is defined by those who have other subtle and frequently overlooked speech problems that can be classified as mild dysarthria. Chad is a perfect example of such a client.

CHAD

Chad was a seven-year-old boy who had no other learning problems other than articulation error. He was enrolled in a regular second-grade classroom where he functioned adequately. Chad was referred to me for help on the R sound on a consultative basis by his regular school-based therapist. The referring therapist reported that Chad's only error was on R. She explained that he could not be stimulated for correct production of R despite more than one year of treatment. When pressed for more information, the referring therapist admitted that he was "a little hard to understand." She assured me, however, that R was his only real error.

Upon examination, I found that Chad was hard to understand when he spoke on unfamiliar topics. His sibilants and L were interdentalized intermittently. He was somewhat hoarse, was aphonic at times and had nasal flaring with slight hypernasality. Chad distorted a variety of vowels slightly, and he omitted whole syllables here and there. He spoke slowly in a monotone and did not project his voice well. His R was distorted. Chad's lips moved asymmetrically throughout conversation, and the jaw appeared stiff and immobile during speech. Chad was quite hesitant to speak, but both his mother and the referring therapist reassured me that I was hearing Chad's typical speech patterns.

What is the difference between what I observed and that which the referring therapist reported? Chad's R distortion was the only "real error" noted by his referring therapist because that was all she was looking for. He had been referred to her initially for an error on R. She was attending to this and nothing else. This therapist was not trained to pay attention to the other minor and inconsistent errors on vowels and syllables that were present, even though these interfered with consistent intelligibility. She ignored his lack of pitch and loudness variations. She was unconcerned about inconsistent tongue-tip placement. She did not see the general oral-motor deficit, and she did not realize that R was a part of a much bigger problem. Chad's real problem was one of mild dysarthria, and his distortion of R was only one manifestation of it.

Chad's story illustrates that a distortion of R can be observed in clients who display other subtle deficits in articulation, voice, resonance and prosody. Generally, these kids can articulate fairly well when they recite one word at a time, so their production of most phonemes may be quite good during an articulation test. Careful analysis of articulation during the demands of rapid conversational speech reveals, however, that their speech is sloppy or muffled. Parents report that these children are hard to understand and that they mumble when they talk. They are accused of not trying to say R correctly. Further, a "wet" or "slushy" quality may be reported due to excessive saliva accumulating in the mouth.

Careful analysis of articulation reveals that these children usually have one or more of the following additional speech patterns:

- Intermittent L distortion: tongue-tip placement varies, the blade may be used
- Intermittent sibilant distortion: midline air stream varies in position
- Intermittent lateralization on lingua-alveolar sounds—T, D, N, L, S, Z
- Slight distortion of other consonants
- Slight vowel distortion, especially on multisyllabic words
- Irregular and somewhat rapid rate: too fast for oral abilities
- Slightly poor volume control: somewhat too loud, quiet or irregular
- Aperiodic slight hypernasality: on the vowels, or as a syllable substitute
- Slight monotone or other intonation differences
- Aperiodic consonant cluster reduction
- Variations in the ability to retain syllables in multisyllabic words

The problems listed above that occur alongside an R distortion often are overlooked because most speech and language pathologists have not been taught to recognize mild dysarthria. Very little training has been offered regarding minor differences in prosody, resonance and rate, and inconsistent errors on consonants and vowels are treated as inconsequential. The popular notion is that these sounds are emerging and that the client's speech is a little immature. Although it is true that these phonemes and prosodic features are emerging, they are *not* immature; they are different and distorted. Without this correct view, such a client's R sound may be the only error considered for remediation because it is the only feature that draws his therapist's attention. In fact, without the distortion of R, the child may not even be referred for evaluation nor qualify for treatment.

Why do these phoneme and prosodic errors go unrecognized? First, most speech and language pathologists have been trained to think first and foremost about blatant consonant errors. Minor and inconsistent errors on the vowels and the prosodic features usually are completely ignored. Second, slight distortion on most other consonants goes unnoticed because the range of acceptability for their production is quite broad. For example, even a severe distortion of B can be completely overlooked because it can be recognized as B and its distortion does not interfere with intelligibility. A phoneme like B has a broad *range of acceptability* and we accept many variations of this sound as correct and within the normal range. The R sound is very different, however. Even a slight distortion causes R to stand out as an error because its range of acceptability is quite narrow. There is only one good R sound. Beyond that, all else is distortion. This is what makes R so problematic in childhood.

Mild dysarthria is, in my experience, a very common occurrence in the population of clients with longterm persistent R distortion. Their dysarthria is very subtle in nature, but significant enough to impact speech as described above. This is the client who seems resistant to R therapy because his distortion of R is a manifestation of his overall mild dysarthric pattern. Treatment that focuses solely on the production of R will be met with limited success in many of these cases because restricted oral-motor and speech skills inhibit the client's ability to learn R. He is not ready. The work is too subtle. Treatment for such a client must address prosodic elements, oral-motor skills, auditory discrimination of a wide range of speech features, vowels, R and any other consonants that are impacted. Working on R itself may be the foundation of the treatment program, and may be the reason the client is enrolled. But therapy may only succeed when the other aspects of the real problem are addressed.

Speech and language pathologists are asked to take a second, very discriminating look at their R clients to determine if any fit this category. Be very picky in this assessment, and do not gloss over minor characteristics that may seem unimportant at first glance. Document every type of error these clients make, and see the bigger picture. Your therapy will improve significantly when you do because it will address the specific causes of the R distortion. Further, these clients may qualify for treatment at a younger age with more thorough documentation of the entire problem.

Category 3: Distortion of R with No Oral-Motor Deficit

Distortion of R also can occur alone amidst an otherwise intact speech-production system. This third category is the one that bothers the greatest number of therapists. When R truly is the client's only speech sound distortion, it means that he simply has not figured out how to position the jaw, lips and tongue correctly for R alone. General oral-motor skills are good, prosodic features are well-developed and all other phonemes are well-formed. Intelligibility can be very high. This client simply has settled on incorrect oral movements or positions for R, and R is the only sound produced in an incorrect way. The client's incorrect oral-movement pattern for production of R is his habit. Treatment is designed to break this habit while establishing new correct movement patterns.

An inability to achieve R when it is the only speech error usually has one of two manifestations. Either the client cannot achieve a correct target position and can produce no correct R sounds, or the client has trouble with the gliding movements around R.

PROBLEMS WITH THE APEX OF MOVEMENT

The distortion of R with an otherwise intact speech production system can occur at the apex position itself, and the most common problem concerns a difference in how the back of the tongue is positioned during production of the Back R. As discussed in the last chapter, proper Back R is made as the back-lateral margins stabilize at the molars while the middle back tenses upward slightly without touching the palates. Clients who fit this category usually attempt R by positioning the tongue in the opposite way. They depress, lower or leave lax the back-lateral margins of the tongue, and they elevate the middle section of the back.

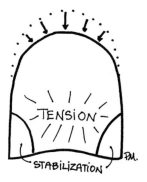

Fig. 2. Tongue position for the correct Back R. Notice that the back-lateral margins are high and stable and that the middle back is tense.

Fig. 2.1. Tongue position for the distorted Back R. Notice that the middle back is very high and the lateral back margins are low and lax.

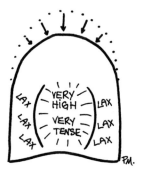

This aberrant apex position causes the classic R distortion that an experienced therapist can recognize immediately as one that will not be outgrown once habituated. It is one of the most difficult of all the minor articulation errors to remediate because of the subtle oral-movement problem at its core. The difference between this position and that required for a perfect R sound can be nearly impossible to perceive for many clients. In fact, many speech and language pathologists even have difficulty perceiving this difference at first. The following exercise will help the reader understand this exceptionally common error.

EXERCISE 2.1
LEARN TO PRODUCE A CLASSIC BACK R DISTORTION

You can learn to produce the classic Back R distortion by working with the lateral lisp. Produce a bilateral lisp on S. Make sure you make it by pressing the middle of your tongue up against the palate. Notice that the middle of your tongue is pressing firmly upward and that the sides of the tongue are low. Low sides allow the air stream to escape laterally. Hold this position firmly so you can feel the articulation of the middle of the tongue against the roof of the mouth well. Now, lower the overall tongue position slightly away from the palate while maintaining the strong upward push of the tongue's middle. Say R without altering the position. Keep the tongue's middle high. Do you hear the sound that results? This is the classic distortion of R caused by elevation of the tongue's middle back while the sides remain low.

EXERCISE 2.2
ALTERNATE BETWEEN CORRECT BACK R AND THE CLASSIC BACK R DISTORTION

[This exercise can be done only if you know how to produce a correct Back R as well as the Classic R Distortion described in the exercise above.] Produce a correct Back R and then a Classic Back R Distortion. Alternate them back and forth. Attend to the differences of position and tension in the back of the tongue.

The great tragedy of the Classis R Distortion is that many speech and language pathologists teach their clients to make a Back R by "lifting up the back of the tongue." This is an incorrect description of the movement necessary to achieve the Back R. It may be an adequate description for easy clients, but it will end in disaster for the difficult ones. It will cause the Classic Distortion to occur! Correct articulation of the Back R is made through differential control of the middle back from the lateral backs of the tongue. With a gross description to "lift the back of the tongue," the difficult client usually does one of two things. He either lifts the entire back of the tongue or he lifts the middle back alone. Either will cause distortion. A client who has not developed the back of the tongue will continue to lift the back to no avail and his therapy will end in failure. This client needs to be taught how to differentially control the middle from side backs. To make a Back R, the client needs to learn to stabilize the back-lateral margins, and then to elevate and tense the middle at the same time. Or he needs to learn a Tip R.

PROBLEMS WITH ON-GLIDE AND OFF-GLIDE MOVEMENTS

Many longterm R clients actually can achieve correct apex position for R and can pronounce an adequate R sound with either a Tip R or a Back R position. The problem is that their phoneme continues to sound distorted because the movements required for the on-glide or off-glide are incorrect. Improper on-glide or off-glide movements cause other sounds to be added around the basic R sound. These other sounds cause R to sound distorted, although the correct acoustic quality of R is present in the utterance. Referring therapists usually describe these clients in the following ways:

- "He can say R—at least, I think he's saying it okay."
- "He does funny things."
- "He's doing something wrong."
- "It doesn't always sound good."
- "I don't know if I'm hearing it right."
- "He's just not getting anywhere."
- "He says some things right, but not always."

The referring therapist is trying to say that she hears an acoustically correct R sound buried in the midst of distortion caused by incorrect on-glide and off-glide movements. She also means that the acceptability of the sound varies from one trial to the next, depending upon what the client actually does during each individual gliding movement. These gliding alterations are always idiosyncratic ones. In fact, there probably are as many ways to distort the on-glide or off-glide of R as there are clients who do this. However, several patterns are noted most frequently:

- *Adding Labial Stridency:* Some client produce a V-like sound just before, just after or simultaneously with a correct R. The result is a V-and-R sound for R. For example, a client might produce *radio* as *vradio* or *rvadio*. These could be classified as a VR-for-R or an RV-for-R substitution, but the overall acoustic effect is more one of distortion than substitution. The client is adding inappropriate labio-dental movement and stridency to the on-glide or off-glide of R.
- *Adding Labial Gliding:* Some clients produce a W-like sound just after a correct R. The result is a RW sound for R. For example, the client might produce *run* as *rwun*. The client is adding inappropriate labial movement to the off-glide. Often this is a stage that occurs after the classic W-for-R substitution and before true R is settled. Although minor in scope, many clients get stuck with this pattern if it is not addressed directly, and the result is lifelong unusual R distortion.

- *Adding Liquid Gliding to the Off-glide:* Many clients produce an L-like sound on the off-glide after producing an acoustically correct R sound. For example, a client might produce *rabbit* as *rlabbit*. Usually these clients can produce a decent R in the final position but cannot produce R without this added sound in the initial position because the error occurs on the off-glide. The added sound is not usually a true L sound. Instead, it too is a distortion and often a flop. As a result, the listener's ear picks up this error as a distortion to the basic R sound, but it is not. It is a distorted L sound that has been added to R's off-glide, and that is embedded between R and the following vowel.

These are the most common distortions of R encountered on a regular basis, but there are other odd differences that appear in individual cases. Distortion errors are the result of unstable or incorrect jaw, lip or tongue movements and positions. The speech and language pathologist must be vigilant in listening to these distortions in order to hear them correctly. And she must carefully study the oral movements made during production of the error in order to determine what the incorrect movements are and whether they are added to the on-glide, the off-glide or the apex of speech movement.

A Continuum of R Distortion

It is proposed that the longterm persistent R distortion occurs on a continuum of oral-motor deficit. On one end of this continuum are those clients with pervasive severe neuromuscular dysfunction. At the other end are clients with no obvious oral-motor deficit. Between these extremes are those clients who demonstrate R distortion as one part of mild dysarthria. My clinical experiences in almost three decades of therapy have taught me that the numbers of clients in each category are spread over the classic bell-shaped curve, with most clients scoring in the middle category. The diagram below summarizes this idea. Please realize that this diagram represents the oral-motor deficits found in clients with persistent R distortion and not those with substitution or omission. Also please recognize that this is an impression formed after thirty years of clinical study.

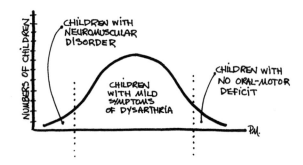

Fig. 2.2 Distortion of R appears to occur on a continuum of oral-motor deficit.

A Deeper View of Oral Movement

Any distortion of R is the result of absent, problematic or poorly-timed jaw, lip, tongue or velar movements. These are the problems that are seen in clients with R distortion, and these are the things that need fixing in successful R therapy. An exercise designed to help readers understand these concepts is included in each section below. All these factors are taken into consideration as we discuss treatment techniques in subsequent chapters.

The Jaw's Impact on R

From its hinge at the temporomandibular joint, the jaw is designed to move in the following ways: up, down, left, right, forward, back and in rotation in all directions. For speech, it moves subtly in all these directions, but stays relatively high near the neutral position so that the tongue can make consistent contact with the palate and the lips can approximate together. The neutral position of the jaw is its position at rest. At rest, the lips are closed, giving the appearance that the upper and lower teeth are touching. This is not true. In the neutral position at rest, the jaw sits slightly low so that the upper and lower molars are near one another but not touching. The jaw moves in a finely graded and restricted range around this position for speech.

Traditional articulation evaluation and treatment procedures pay almost no attention to jaw movement problems in speech sound error, including errors on R. However, my observations of oral-motor skills in hundreds of clients with longterm persistent R distortion have revealed that jaw movement and position often is incorrect, and that these differences can contribute significantly to R distortion. The following are noted:

- The jaw may be positioned too high or low in target position for R.
- The jaw may fail to stabilize appropriately to accommodate good tongue position for R.
- The jaw may lateralize, protrude or retract during the on-glide or off-glide phases of R.
- Jaw movements may be poorly synchronized with lip, tongue or velar movements.
- Jaw movements may be too gross to accommodate the refined tongue movements needed for R.
- In cases of severe neuromuscular disorder with spasticity, the jaw may be nearly immobile during speech.

Each of these movement differences cause R to be distorted unless other parts of the oral mechanism compensate for them. Successful R therapy includes procedures to analyze and treat incorrect jaw movements during production of the sound in various speech contexts. The following exercise is designed to bring clarity on these patterns.

EXERCISE 2.3
Discover the Effects of Jaw Position on R Production

Prolong an isolated R for fifteen seconds while moving the jaw into undesirable positions. Listen to the acoustic changes on R that result. For example, move the jaw upward so high that the mouth actually closes. Then move it downward as far as it will go so that the mouth is fully open. Move the jaw far to the left and right, and then protrude and retract it as far as you can.

What happens to the acoustic quality of R as you make these height and alignment changes in your jaw position? You should discover that the acoustic quality of R changes or distorts. The change might be slight, moderate or severe, depending on how much your tongue and lip positions change with the jaw position difference. Experiment with these inappropriate movements for a few moments until you are sure you hear the changes. Then focus on the position your jaw assumes when you speak your "perfect R."

The Lips' Impact on R

The lips round, retract, separate and come back together during speech. During production of R, the lips sometimes round and sometimes retract slightly depending upon how the jaw and tongue are placed. The lips help shape the sound of R once the jaw and tongue position are set. When R is distorted, lip position often is poorly coordinated with jaw and tongue movements. Sometimes just the slightest change to lip position will help the acoustic quality of R to snap into position. Successful R therapy includes techniques to position the lips to advantage for good R resonance. The following exercise is designed to bring clarity on this idea.

EXERCISE 2.4
Discover the Effects of Lip Position on R Productions

Produce an isolated R in the Tip or Back position, and prolong it while you alter lip position. Pucker the lips forward slightly, and then pucker them firmly so that the lips nearly close. What happens to your R? Now, retract the lips all the way back into a tight smiling position. How is R different now? Also, prolong an isolated R as you lift the upper lip into a sneer and when you lower the bottom lip away from the teeth.

How does the acoustic quality of R change as your lip positions change? Does it change in each case? Do you feel the associated changes in tongue position that occur as you alter lip position and tension? Can you hear the distortion that occurs as a result? Train your ear to identify the sometimes slight, sometimes drastic alterations in sound quality that occur as lip position changes.

The Tongue's Impact on Tip R and Back R

While jaw and lip position are important for correct R production, the most critical oral movements involve tongue position. Most clients with longterm persistent R distortion have great difficulty getting the tongue into a correct position, and this is the very thing that prevents them from attaining an adequate R. Both the Tip R and the Back R become significantly distorted when the tongue does not achieve its correct position. Thus, successful articulation therapy for a correct R focuses significant attention on movement and position of the tongue. The following exercises are designed to bring clarity on this foundational idea.

EXERCISE 2.5
Discover the Effect of Tongue Position Changes on Tip R

Prolong an isolated R sound using the Tip R position. Then alter the tongue in several ways and note the acoustic changes:

1. Prevent the tip from going high enough.
2. Make the tip go up in the front but fail to scoop back.
3. Make the tip elevate toward one side or the other in the back.
4. Curl the tip down instead of up.
5. Curl the tip upward outside the mouth.
6. Curl the tip up, but allow the tongue to be lax.
7. Make the tip go too high and too far back into the oropharynx.
8. Lift the middle of the tongue along with the tip.

EXERCISE 2.6
Discover the Effect of Tongue Position Changes on Back R Productions

Prolong an isolated R sound using the Back R position. Then experiment with the following position changes and note the acoustic results:

1. Make the lateral backs go too high.
2. Do not lift the lateral margins high enough.
3. Elevate the middle back too high.
4. Assume a correct position, but allow the tongue to be too lax.

The Velum's Impact on R

Phoneme R becomes severely distorted when upward movement of the velum is absent or inadequate in some way, or when movement of the velum is poorly synchronized with jaw, lip and tongue movements. These errors cause sound to escape through the nasal passageways with resultant hypernasality on R. Successful R therapy always includes procedures to diagnose and treat velar movement problems when hypernasality is present. Adequate control of the velum for differential oral and nasal production of sound is critical for successful R production. Therefore, it needs to be carefully considered.

EXERCISE 2.7
Discover the Effect of Velopharyngeal Change on R Production

It is difficult to alter velar position purposefully, but you can do so with a little instruction. First, say the Ng sound as in the word *sing*. This sound will drive your voice through the nose. Now say an isolated R sound in the same way, with the velum lowered and the sound driving through your nose. The sound you make should not be much different from Ng. This is the distortion of R that is heard when the velar mechanism is impacted by neuromuscular disorder or velopharyngeal inadequacy. It also is heard among some clients purely as a habitual production pattern when the velopharyngeal mechanism functions perfectly well.

Other Movement Impacts on R
We have described the primary movement problems associated with R distortion. However, there are a few others that are noted occasionally. Try these yourself. They include:

- Inhalation instead of exhalation during R production
- Production of a voiceless instead of a voiced sound during R production
- Production of a velar fricative for R while in correct position
- Production of a lateral velar fricative for R while in correct position

Make It Just Right
A correct production of R occurs when oral movements and positions are just right. The essential oral-motor patterns are the same for all speakers, although the size and shape of each individual mouth and its component parts will dictate slight changes here and there. We could make an analogy to the hand to explain this difference. Take the movements necessary to make a fist, for example. No two fists will look exactly the same, because every person's hand is shaped a little differently from everyone else. But the basic movement patterns needed to move into the fist position and the final position itself will be essentially the same for every person. In production of R, a wide mouth with a low palate requires an oral position that may be slightly different than that needed for a narrow mouth with a high palate. However, the essential movements and positions needed to produce R are the same for all speakers. Only a severe structural difference due to malformation, disease or injury would necessitate an oral-movement position that was completely different than the norm.

Clients rely upon us to help them discern and produce a correct R phoneme. Therefore, all speech and language pathologists should take time to work through the exercises in this chapter so that subtle variations on R can be learned. The exercises in this chapter may be difficult for some readers to do at first. With time and practice, however, most therapists will be able to control the fine differences in jaw, lip, tongue and velar movements that result in distortion. Practice with the exercises will help the reader learn to hear the correct acoustic quality of the perfect R sound, and to discriminate between it and all other variations. These skills are necessary for remediation of R. Without it, the professional speech and language pathologist will be completely lacking in the very skills that are the basis of remediation. One can further enrich this experience by practicing all the incorrect R sounds produced by clients, ESL speakers and little children who are learning R. I do this. I never pass up an opportunity to imitate an R that is slightly outside of the range of normal. Such work broadens one's direct experience with R and helps at all levels of treatment.

— *Summary* —

- Problems with the R sound occur in three basic ways: by omission, substitution, or distortion.

- Omission and substitution of R are the most common forms of misarticulation in normal development. They are the easiest to change because there are no incorrect oral-motor patterns to alter.

- The W-for-R substitution is so common in speech sound acquisition that it is expected amongst young children and is classified as a developmental error. The W-for-R substitution is a stop on the path of normal development.

- The distorted R is a deviant pattern that is the most difficult one to change. It represents a deviation from the normal path. This is the R that is most resistant to remediation because incorrect oral-movement patterns must be inhibited while new patterns are acquired.

- Clients with R distortion come in three basic types: those with severe, those with mild, and those with no oral-motor dysfunction. It is proposed that these three types occur on a continuum from mild-to-severe oral-motor dysfunction.

- The distortion of R is caused by incorrect jaw, lip, tongue or velar movements and positions. Some distortions are the result of sound being added to the basic R sound.

- Phoneme R is made correctly only when jaw, lip, tongue and velar movements are just right. These positions are the same generally for all people. However, slight variations are noted as size and shape of the oral mechanism differ from person to person.

- Speech and language pathologists should become proficient in identifying how alterations in jaw, lip, tongue and velar movements change the acoustic quality of the R sound. The ability to understand oral movement to a high level of skill is required for the professional speech and language pathologist to be effective in treatment of R misarticulation.

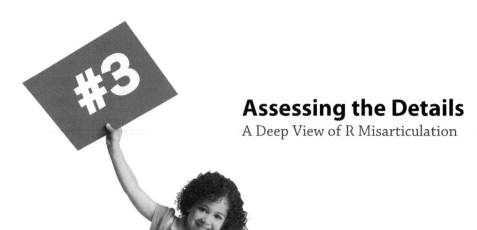

Assessing the Details
A Deep View of R Misarticulation

The course of treatment for the misarticulated R begins, of course, with assessment. The purpose of the assessment is to identify the problem, pinpoint possible causes and design an initial treatment plan. This is the time to dig deeply into the cause and nature of the misarticulated R so that the client's time in treatment can be maximized. An assessment of R should include at least the following:

- Background investigation
- Conversational speech sample
- Articulation testing
- Imitation of the distortion
- Examination of oral structure
- Examination of oral-motor skills
- Production of the "very best" R
- Response to selected treatment techniques
- Discussion of purpose
- Commitment to therapy

Each of these components is described below along with introductory suggestions about treatment. Greater discussion of treatment techniques will continue in the next and subsequent chapters.

The Background Investigation
The goal of the background investigation is to identify factors that have contributed to or that still may be contributing to the R problem. The background check should include standard questions about speech, language and general development, including cognitive development. It also should explore issues regarding hearing, illness, hospitalization, surgery, education and family background. Specific attention should be given to history of speech, language or feeding delay, prior speech-therapy services, and medical issues related to the mouth, e.g., surgery, orthodontia, velopharyngeal concerns, and so forth. Questions also

should be asked about past or present oral habits, such as thumb or pacifier sucking, and attempts to reduce or eliminate them. The background assessment allows the speech and language pathologist to understand how the problematic R fits into the client's overall life situation. This broad view helps determine the course of treatment. Background information is put together with other data to make decisions regarding the plan of treatment and its projected outcome. Specific examples of background influences on the treatment of R are described in the case studies presented in chapter 4.

Conversational Speech Sample

The conversational speech sample is one of the most important aspects of the entire initial examination. Much useful information can be gained, including data on articulation, voice, prosody, and intelligibility. A general dialogue also is used to build rapport between therapist and client. The examiner should lead the conversation into areas of interest for the client so that he will begin to think more about what he is saying and less about how he is saying it. If the client appears to be trying to produce his best R during the talk, ask him to relax and not to try so hard. Ask him to speak the way he always does with his friends when he is not trying to sound better. Let him know that you do not care how he sounds during this first meeting. Tell him that you want to hear his natural speech. The average client will begin to show you his habitual speech sometime during the session. Shy or self-conscious clients may not open up and speak freely for some time, so do not fret if you do not get this perspective right away. But make sure you get it sometime early in treatment. Begin to take note of overall speaking skill once the client demonstrates a fairly natural speech pattern. Ask the client to tell you his name, address and phone number, etc., as a way to hear his natural speech before he is ready to open up. Also, ask him to count to fifty and recite the alphabet. These are simple ways to get a spontaneous speech sample without having a real conversation.

- *Articulation:* Use the conversational speech sample to determine if R is the only problem or if there are errors on other sounds. Be very picky in this regard. Pay particular attention to the client's production of the other glides and the vowels. Note even slight deviations on any of them. Also note minor deviations on other consonants, and carefully watch for signs of interdentalization and lateralization. Determine if R is the only deviated phoneme or if there is a broader problem. Subtle differences on other sounds are very important when assessing an R problem. Be quite honest with yourself and ask, "Am I hearing only an R problem, or is there more to this?"
- *Voice and Prosody:* Observe pitch, quality, resonance, strength, intensity and duration of voice during conversation. Also observe rate, rhythm, stress and intonation. Does the child seem to talk too fast for his articulation ability? Does he sound jerky or aphonic? Is he hyper- or hyponasal? Is he struggling to be loud enough, or is he too loud for the situation? Does he produce a glottal fry on R?
- *Intelligibility:* Pay particular attention to the client's ability to attain and maintain intelligibility in rapid conversation. Do you find yourself having to listen hard to understand him at times? Do consonants or vowels disappear or change periodically?

Do blends reduce intermittently? Do syllables drop out at times? Is intelligibility consistent, or does it fluctuate? Does the child mumble? Does he sound muffled? Is he sloppy? Could you understand him if there was other noise or conversation in the room? How would he sound if he were standing in front of a class and speaking this way? Would this be good oration?

Articulation Test

Formal articulation testing is initiated in order to specify phoneme errors made on word productions. Words can be elicited by spontaneous means or through imitations. For spontaneous productions consider using picture- or object-naming tasks, answers to questions or fill-in-the-blank statements.

COMPLETE ASSESSMENT

A complete assessment of articulation skill is necessary when conversational speech sampling reveals deviations in other phonemes besides R. The complete assessment will help identify all present speech sound errors, including that on R. Any standard articulation test, whether professionally published or homemade, will do. Make sure to test the vowels and diphthongs as well as all the consonants and clusters. Identify any and all deviations however slight, and note how the sounds are deviated and to what degree. For example, mark an interdentalized sibilant as such, and do not simply mark it as D for "distorted." Such detail will help determine your course of treatment.

PARTIAL ASSESSMENT

A partial assessment may be sufficient if initial conversational speech sampling has revealed that R truly is the only error phoneme. Partial assessments can be used freely when working with older children who obviously have an otherwise intact expressive speech sound system. Be warned: Time and again, slight problems on other phonemes will be discovered later in therapy when the initial complete articulation assessment is omitted. Remember that most children, even older ones, with a longterm persistent R distortion usually have subtle errors on other phonemes. A partial assessment may not reveal these.

DEEP TEST

After the complete or partial assessment of articulation ability has been completed, it is important to go one step further to understand the nature of the R problem by initiating a deep test. The purpose of the deep test of R is to give the examiner time to hear the client's R in a wide variety of speech contexts. Ask the client to name pictures or imitate words that contain R in the initial, medial and final position of words, before and after most of the vowels and diphthongs, and in blends. The goal of the deep test is to determine how R is treated in a wide variety of coarticulated conditions. Determine whether R is omitted, substituted or distorted in each. Pay very careful attention if R is pronounced correctly in some contexts and incorrectly in others. Correct productions, if any, will comprise the beginning points in treatment. Make it your mission to find them! Without them, treatment begins from scratch. The tables below offer several good sets of words for deep testing.

The reader will observe that there are dozens of words that could be tested in the deep-test analysis. Producing such a great number of such words when R clearly is in error can be embarrassing to a client during an assessment. Since it is more important to establish rapport than it is to completely test the R misarticulation early in treatment, it is not important that all these words be tested during the first session. The intake examiner simply can spot check a few selected words to gain an overview of the errors. Then the deep-test words can be spread casually over the first several weeks of therapy. This will masquerade the test and make it seem less confrontational or embarrassing.

SAMPLE WORDS TO TEST CONSONANTAL R

/ri/	reap, reach
/rɪ/	rid, rich
/re/	rate, raven
/rɛ/	red, rend
/ræ/	rat, racoon
/ru/	room, roost
/rʊ/	rook, roof
/ro/	rope, Rome
/rɔ/	raw, raucous
/rɑ/	rock, rod
/rʌ/	rug, rum

SAMPLE WORDS TO TEST VOCALIC R

/ɝ/	term
/ɚ/	utter
/iɚ/	tear
/uɚ/	tour
/oɚ/	store
/ɑɚ/	star
/ɑiɚ/	tire
/ɑuɚ/	tower
/ɔiɚ/	foyer
/eiɚ/	stair

SAMPLE WORDS TO TEST CONSONANTAL R IN BLENDS

/pr/	prove, pride
/br/	brown, brave
/tr/	truck, train
/dr/	drum, dream
/kr/	crack, cream

/gr/	green, grass
/str/	street, strike
/skr/	scratch, scream
/ʃr/	shriek, shred
/θr/	throw, thrash

SAMPLE WORDS TO TEST VOCALIC R IN BLENDS

vocalic R blend	word samples
with /m/	term, form, farm
with /n/	burn, barn, born
with /l/	curl, girl, world
with /s/	purse, horse, tires
with /z/	doors, purrs, cars
with /p/	warp, chirp, carp
with /b/	orb, perturb, "carb"
with /t/	hurt, abort, cart
with /d/	word, Ford, bard
with /k/	park, Turk, pork
with /g/	iceberg, Pittsburgh
with /dʒ/	purge, George, large
with /st/	burst, first
with /θ/	Garth, earth

Very Best R

Further information is gained about a client's production of R when we ask him to produce his very best R. We ask our client to make this sound after we have gained a sample of the R sound that he habitually uses in conversational speech. We want to see what he does when he's really trying to perform his best. This step is especially necessary when a client has been in prior speech therapy and phoneme R was addressed. The best production will reveal what the client has been taught in prior therapies. It will inform us whether prior therapy was geared toward a Tip R or a Back R, and whether it tended toward a Consonantal R or a Vocalic R. It also will reveal whether these aspects of R production even were considered in therapy.

The production of the very best R also shows us what the client thinks he is supposed to do, and it lets us see how much control he actually has over his speech mechanism. The client's prior experiences become even more apparent when we ask him to explain to us what he is doing to make his very best R sound. The vocabulary he uses and the description he makes lets us know how much he actually knows about his problem and the ways to fix it.

Therapy fails when we try to add new patterns on top of old bad habits learned during years of unproductive R therapy. These problems will be revealed when a client is asked to produce his very best R. Some clients have been asked to try so many different ways to achieve an R sound that all the methods they have been introduced to have become a jumble in their minds. Adding new techniques on top of this mess only makes the situation worse. Ideally, we search for the original mistake the client was making before he tried to change it. This is not to say that all prior therapy was bad. But the essence of designing a good treatment program is to provide exactly what the client needs. You want to eliminate those habits and patterns that don't contribute to positive growth. Usually this means getting down to the original error. The original error demonstrates the actual trouble the client had in learning R in the first place.

Imitation of the Distortion
The diagnosis of an R distortion includes procedures for determining exactly what the client is doing wrong. Because it is almost impossible to see inside the mouth during R production, the best way to accomplish this is for the therapist to imitate the client's incorrect production. The imitation of the client's distorted R allows the examiner to feel the movement and position problem. In my work with practicing therapists across North America, I have found few who utilize this type of assessment. When asked, "Can you make the sound just as your client does?" most therapists respond that they cannot. This is a shame. An imitation of the client's incorrect production is an extremely useful part of assessment. It instructs the examining therapist precisely about what the client is doing wrong. It can be more valuable than any other piece of the assessment.

Imitating the client exactly can be difficult to do. In fact, it can be as hard for us to imitate a client's incorrect production as it is for him to imitate our correct one. But time spent trying to imitate the client exactly is well worth the effort. To do so, one must develop enough oral skill to mimic a wide variety of incorrect R sounds. Perhaps the easiest way to imitate a client is to do so in a synchronistic manner. This means to produce an R while the client does. Ask the client to prolong his sound. This allows you time to hear it and play around with your own sound to find the match. This can take a while because there are about as many ways to distort R as there are clients who distort it. Each client seems to have his own idiosyncratic or signature distortion.

An exact imitation of a client's distortion may be unobtainable during the first treatment session. But the skill can come outside of therapy while practicing alone if you have paid very close attention and can recall the sound later. Play with various ways of producing the R sound until you chance upon the one the client produces. Then repeat that sound until you master it. Then begin to bend the sound ever so slightly from that position until you reach an acoustically correct one. This experimentation will teach you a great deal about training your client.

Please note that being able to produce an exact copy of a client's incorrect production is not a prerequisite to therapy. One can still proceed without it. In fact, sometimes clients make oral movements in such unusual ways that it is impossible for us to replicate their R distortion for some time. It can take weeks to figure out how a particular client is making his distorted R sound. In such cases, one can move ahead, but the drive to understand the client's misarticulation through imitation of him should not stop. Eventually the sound will be analyzed correctly. The oral-movement problem becomes suddenly clear. The treatment process becomes more fruitful after that because the work can be tailored exactly to the client's oral movement needs.

There is an additional benefit to this process. Learning to imitate the wide variety of R distortions our clients make helps us become better assessors of incorrect R sounds. Through the years, our own oral-motor and related auditory discrimination skills for slight distortions of R improve significantly and, as a result, we become better teachers of the sound.

The Examination of Oral Structure

A professional speech and language evaluation always includes an examination of oral structure. The oral-structure exam includes a visual inspection of the face, nose, lips, cheeks, jaw, hard and soft palates, tongue, teeth, gums, floor of the mouth and oropharynx. The size and shape of bony tissues and muscles are inspected, along with the color and condition of the skin. Deviations are noted.

It is not the purpose of this book to explain the examination of oral structure. Every speech and language pathology student learns it in school. Instead, we shall focus on the oral-structure problems frequently noted in R misarticulation. There has been no stellar research on the relationship between the persistent R distortion and oral structure. However, my clinical observations of many hundreds of client's with longterm persistent R distortions have indicated several specific characteristics that are noteworthy because of their high frequency of occurrence in clients with longterm persistent R distortion. In no specific order these include:

- Small oral cavity
- Small jaw
- Small tongue
- Narrow tongue
- Restricting lingua frenum
- High arched palate
- Large tongue
- Narrow palate
- Deep oropharynx
- Malocclusion
- Slow emergence of the molars

Obviously, there is no one-to-one relationship between these characteristics and distortion of R. Not every child with these characteristics will have a distorted R, and clearly these characteristics do not cause an R distortion. These characteristics are noted often in cases of longterm persistent R distortion. Why? The answer is unknown. Perhaps variations in the size and shape of the oral cavity prevent some children from learning R during the normal time. Perhaps these children are less able to adapt to the specifics of their oral shape than other children. Or perhaps these children are the ones who have a combination of three deficient areas: oral-structure differences, poor auditory discrimination skills and poor oral-motor control. This combination of problems certainly contributes negatively to speech learning. Since R is one of the most difficult phonemes to learn, it may be natural for these children to have difficulty learning it.

The purpose of the examination of oral structure is to determine if there are factors that may have contributed to the R problem or that hinder current development. A thorough examination of oral structure allows one to make important decisions about treatment. The following notes are offered as a short summary of the problems caused by the oral characteristics listed above. These notes are not meant to suggest a causative relationship between these characteristics and a distorted R production. Every case is different. In some cases, these characteristics have been shown to interfere with the emergence of a correct R production.

- *Small oral cavity:* A small oral cavity should not interfere with the correct acoustic quality of the R sound. However, it can make the voice sound high in pitch and it can make can make it difficult for some clients to achieve the full round quality of the R sound. Since nothing will be done about a small oral cavity in most cases, therapy must work around it. The best acoustic quality possible should be the goal.
- *Small jaw:* A small jaw is usually associated with a small tongue. The small tongue can cause problems as described below.
- *Small tongue:* The small tongue can be unable to stretch its tip toward the back to make a Tip R. The Back R is a better option for treatment.
- *Narrow tongue:* The narrow tongue can interfere with the stretch and elevation of the tongue's lateral margins toward the palate necessary to produce a Back R. The Tip R is a better option.
- *Restricting lingua frenum:* The restricting lingua frenum is the most devastating oral-structure problem that can interfere with R production. The restricting lingua frenum prevents the tip from stretching up and curling back to form a Tip R. It should not interfere with a Back R. Yet, since the Back R is much more difficult to learn, the client with a restricting lingua frenum and slight oral-movement problems can be left without the ability to learn either R sound. Referral for lingua frenectomy may be a necessary component of treatment. Speech therapy can commence after surgery, and the Tip R should be targeted.
- *High arched palate:* The high arched palate can interfere with a client's ability to achieve a correct acoustic quality for R even when the tongue is correctly placed. The client with a high arched palate has an oral-resonance chamber that is shaped differently than most. He must learn to adjust his tongue position to fit his personal arch shape. Tongue position may have to be higher, more posterior or more anterior than the average in order to attain the sound. When orthodontic devices spread the upper or lower dental arches, changes in the acoustic quality of R can be expected and adjustments to position will be necessary to achieve the correct acoustic quality. Many children accomplish this change on their own. However, children who are currently or who previously were enrolled in articulation therapy may need professional assistance for a short period.

- *Large tongue:* The tongue that is too large for the mouth can be a problem for R and many other phonemes. If the tongue is too large—and not simply low in tone; thus, large in appearance—it will protrude from the mouth. A Tip R will be nearly impossible to achieve since the excursion from outside the mouth to the velum may be too far for the tongue to travel in rapid speech. The Back R should be elected. The Back R should be achievable, barring other problems.
- *Narrow palate:* A palate can be too narrow to accommodate a tongue of adequate proportion. As such, the tongue can be generally delayed in motor development, and R and other phonemes can be affected. The Tip R may be a better option in these cases.
- *Deep oropharynx:* The deep oropharynx can make it difficult to achieve a correct acoustic quality for R. Either R can be attempted as each has equal opportunity for success.
- *Malocclusion:* In general, a malocclusion by itself should not affect the emergence of R. However, a malocclusion often is caused by oral habits, such as thumbsucking, nail biting and the like. Oral habits often have a negative effect on oral-motor development and control. It is the aberrant oral-movement patterns that impact the emergence of R. In the best of circumstances, the oral habit is eliminated prior to or during the course of R treatment and a correct resting position and swallow are developed. Some clients are unable to learn R until their oral habit has been eliminated and correct rest posture and swallowing have been established for one year or more.
- *Slow emergence of the molars:* Years ago Dr. Suzanne Evans Morris suggested that an infant and preschool child's tongue stretches upward to explore each emerging tooth. She suggested that the child does so with those areas of the tongue located immediately below the emerging tooth. Almost all clients coming to R therapy will already have the molars in place. However, it might be that some clients failed to learn R because their molars emerged late. It also may be that the continued absence of the upper molars may make it more difficult for some clients to learn R. They may be unable to stabilize the tongue's back-lateral margins for a Back R production until their molars emerge. The Tip R will be a better choice for these clients.

The Examination of Oral Function

The term *oral function* refers to the movements of the jaw, lips, tongue and velum. Today we call it *oral-motor skills* or *oral movement*. The examination of oral function has gone through a revolution in the past thirty years. When I attended university in the 1970s, we learned to write the following sentence for almost every one of our clients who was without previously diagnosed neurological impairment: "Function of the oral mechanism appeared adequate for speech purposes." In truth, we were virtually clueless about oral function. We did not know what adequate or inadequate oral movement looked like. We talked about "funny-looking kids" and "clumsy mouths," but we rarely wrote these terms in our reports. As a result, every client with an R distortion was viewed as having adequate oral function.

Today our assessment is quite different. With our current understanding of oral-motor skills we can be very clear about oral function as it relates to R misarticulation. The oral-motor exam as it is practiced now includes a systematic observation of jaw, lip and tongue movements during speech, feeding, imitation and oral rest. The oral-motor exam also includes an assessment of oral-tactile sensitivity. A client's ability to move the oral mechanism according to known developmental sequences and normative skills can help us determine whether oral-motor therapy needs to be a part of our treatment for R misarticulation.

It is not the intent of this book to describe the complete oral-motor exam. Readers new to the area of the oral-motor exam and oral-motor therapy are referred to *Oral-Motor Techniques in Articulation and Phonological Therapy* for details. Instead, we shall focus on the particular oral-motor problems seen in clients with persistent R misarticulation.

As discussed in chapter 1, clients with persistent R distortion come in three types: those with severe oral-motor dysfunction, those with subtle oral-motor impairment, and those with incorrect oral-motor habits related to R. Regardless of severity level, all clients have certain oral-movement characteristics that are common when R is distorted. These characteristics appear on a continuum of mild to severe, including one or more of the following:

- Poor differentiation of tongue from jaw and lip movements
- Limitations in tongue mobility
- Weakness in the tongue
- Imprecise and uncoordinated tongue movements
- Poor tongue-tip control
- Poor tongue-back control
- Medial retraction of the tongue's back-lateral margins
- Jaw instability
- Hypo- or hypersensitivity
- Reverse or infantile swallow pattern

Such a laundry list could make all clients with R distortion appear severely impaired in oral function! While this is true for clients with obvious neuromuscular disorder, most clients in R therapy demonstrate only slight to mild problems in these areas. These patterns are so subtle that therapists new to the study of oral-motor therapy may not see them at first. Training alongside another therapist more experienced in oral-motor therapy will help identify these characteristics. The minor oral-motor patterns common among most clients with R distortion make moving and positioning the articulators for production of R difficult. Restrictions in tongue mobility make it hard to get the tongue into any of the right positions. Depressed levels of oral sensitivity confuse them on where the tongue is and what it is doing.

Some problems in tongue movement are mind-boggling. For example, when told, "Lift up the back of your tongue," a client may lift the tip and waggle it. When asked to reach with the tongue tip to the back of the mouth, a client might touch it to the front teeth.

Sometimes a client can get the tongue into position one minute but not the next. Sometimes a client will move the jaw, lips, head, eyes, shoulders or even the hands instead of the tongue. At first, even a mirror does not help. Clients with misarticulation of R frequently cannot open the mouth wide enough for us even to tell what the tongue is doing!

If the problems these clients demonstrate in oral control are so blatant, why is R the only sound error they have? The answer is threefold. First, most of these clients do not have problems only with R. Most have a series of problems, as described in chapter 2. Second, these clients have learned other sounds the way all of us do: by happenstance early in speech development. The sound they did not happen to learn, namely R, has to be learned on purpose. It is during this voluntary control of minute oral movements that we see their difficulties. Third, the problems they have in oral control do not show on the speech radar screen, because all other sounds have a much wider range of acceptability. Remember, a B that is grossly distorted still registers as a B, but an R stands out as a distortion even if it is only slightly mispronounced.

The examination of oral function gives us insight into the course of R therapy for every client. It shows us whether or not oral-motor therapy techniques need to be included. It also shows us whether or not R will be addressed. When oral movement is severely impaired, work on R may not be initiated for some time. When oral-motor skills are slightly or moderately impaired, our work on R will proceed, including oral-motor stimulation right from the start. When oral movement is intact and no deviations can be found, therapy can begin to focus upon the production of R immediately.

The Test of Stimulability

Stimulability refers to a client's immediate response and adaptability to selected treatment techniques. During the course of an initial examination, therapists begin to incorporate sample treatment procedures to determine how easily a client makes changes. The stimulability assessment should incorporate several different techniques to facilitate both a Tip R and a Back R. They should be selected from those that would be used early, midway and later in treatment. Try to check a variety. Therapists should be careful not to include too many techniques that will be too difficult for the client. Remember, the purpose of the initial assessment is to determine the nature of the disorder, a course of treatment and to establish rapport with the client. You do not wish to frustrate him. You want to engage him in a process that demonstrates you respect him and that you know what you are doing. Therefore, include several techniques that will be successful and a few that will be challenging. Use his responses to help determine how treatment will progress.

It is important never to show disappointment if the client responds poorly to any of the more challenging procedures being tested during the examination session. Instead, let the client know that you do not expect him to learn R the first day. I like to tell my clients that I want to try "a bunch of weird things that probably won't make any sense to you now." I make light of the odd procedures so that the client can relax and enjoy the ride. Then I carefully observe in order to determine if any of them spark a better R on the first day. Techniques that can be incorporated into this aspect of the examination can be chosen from any of those that are described in later chapters.

The Discussion of Purpose

An important element of the initial assessment is to probe the client's understanding of the problem. A simple question like, "Why did you come here today?" is all that may be needed to learn what the client knows about his speech disorder.

Some children will answer, "Because I can't say R." This is a great answer. It indicates that the client understands the basics: He can't say R, and he has come to you to fix it. Other clients will give answers that indicate that they have no idea why they have come. Some children say, "Teacher said it was my turn," or, "My mom just brought me." Many children shrug their shoulders and mumble, "I don't know." Sometimes this is the truth. Other times it means that the child does not want to reveal his reason. It also can indicate that the client does not know how to answer in a way that will be pleasing to you. No matter the answer, a client's response to this fundamental question informs us how to begin our discussion.

The Commitment

The final piece of information to be obtained during the initial assessment concerns the client's commitment to the process of therapy. Commitment is essential for success. Without it, the process can be doomed. A simple question like, "Do you want to learn R now?" can be used to open this dialogue. Some clients enter the examination session with a commitment already in place. They want to fix their R distortion and are ready to do so. Others aren't really sure, and they have come to see if they want to get involved in this process. Still others clearly do not want to enroll in therapy. The assessment session or a follow-up phone call is the best time to get a commitment from the client. The commitment can be verbal or written, or perhaps even signed in contract form.

The commitment to treatment can be made only by those clients who have the cognitive skills and maturity to understand. Younger children or those with cognitive impairment cannot make this determination, and the commitment must be made by the parents. In public schools, the parent's commitment is cemented with the signing of the Individualized Educational Plan (IEP). In the private sector, parental commitment includes setting up a schedule and arranging payments.

The Results of Assessment

Upon completion of the speech assessment, the examining therapist will have enough information to determine if, when and how therapy should begin. Goals will be set and a general idea about length of treatment will be determined. A brief report can be written and, in the case of a public school, an IEP can be constructed. When the details of assessment are complete, the treatment program can begin. (See appendices for a sample evaluation report.)

— Summary —

- The course of treatment for the misarticulated R begins with assessment. The purpose is to identify the problem, pinpoint possible causes and design a treatment plan.

- The background investigation helps to identify factors that contribute to the R problem.

- The observation of speech in conversation is one of the most important aspects of the initial examination. Much useful information can be gained regarding articulation, voice, prosody, and intelligibility. A conversation also is used to build rapport between therapist and client.

- The articulation test is initiated to specify phoneme errors made on single-word productions. Options include a complete test, a partial test and a deep test. The deep test helps identify contexts in which R is used correctly. If present, these become the starting point of treatment.

- Imitation of the client's incorrect production allows the examiner to feel the movement and position problem. It is a highly valuable tool that helps design precise treatment.

- The examination of oral structure helps identify factors that may have contributed to the R problem in the first place or that may hinder development of R currently.

- The examination of oral-motor skills is a systematic observation of jaw, lip and tongue movements during speech, feeding, imitation and oral rest. It also includes an assessment of oral-tactile sensitivity. A client's ability to move the oral mechanism according to known developmental sequences can help us determine whether oral-motor therapy needs to be part of our treatment for R misarticulation.

- A test of the client's very best R reveals his habitual pattern of R pronunciation. It reveals the effects of prior therapy so that the current evaluator can determine treatment needs.

- The stimulability test helps determine how easily a client makes changes to selected treatment techniques.

- The initial assessment includes questions that probe the client's understanding of the problem and his commitment to the process of treatment. These questions are directed to parents when the client is too young or unable to understand the commitment.

- At the conclusion of the assessment, a report, a treatment plan and/or an IEP can be written. Treatment may commence subsequent to the evaluation and its paperwork.

#4 Achieving the Impossible
Real Work with Real People

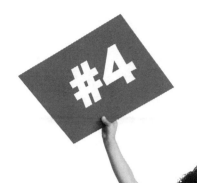

My first R client came to me when I was a student clinician at the University of Illinois. As a young child, Cindy was difficult to understand and had multiple misarticulations. She had succeeded well in school therapy, but was coming to the university at age twelve to fix up her last remaining error on R. I worked with Cindy for about four weeks with no success. Being new to the game, I described muscles and bones to her, trying to be scientific. She could not grasp anything I said. I asked my supervising professor to help me. He spent about three minutes describing how the tongue could form into "mountains and lakes." The girl produced a correct R almost immediately.

Since then I have used this and many other techniques to achieve R, but this first experience taught me several important lessons. Articulation therapy is much more than muscles and bones. Good therapists translate scientific facts into everyday language to fit the imaginations of their clients. Every technique is valuable, no matter its genre. Therapy can be interesting and amusing for both client and instructor. Thirty years of experience teaches therapists much more than textbooks do. And, most importantly, this first lesson taught me that although the treatment of the misarticulated R sometimes is not easy, it is not impossible.

Our techniques come from the fields of oral-motor therapy, traditional articulation therapy, phonological therapy, behavior modification, child development, psychology and more. Such diversity should help make one thing clear: There is no single right way to fix a misarticulated R. Be wary if you have been told that a particular technique is the best thing since Demosthenes for eliciting a correct R. That which makes therapy highly successful for one client may fail miserably for the next. This does not mean that the technique itself is no good. It just means that the technique works selectively with certain clients. All techniques function that way. A therapist's job is to find the right solution for each client so that personal success can be achieved.

Cooking Up a Good Plan
Articulation therapy is an art form based on scientific information. We might compare it to the process a great chef goes through as he creates a new recipe. A recipe contains certain

ingredients. Cake recipes, for example, contain flour, sugar and eggs. To create a new cake recipe, a chef must combine these basic substances with other ingredients in a unique way.

Each individual client in R therapy is like a new cake recipe. The ingredients of R therapy are the stimulation techniques we follow to facilitate the emergence of the sound, and the activities that engage our clients to be interested and motivated. Successful R therapy requires that the ingredients of treatment change in type, amount and sequence for each client. We chose procedures A, B and C for one, and methods X, Y and Z for another. And a different combination for a third. These choices are made during the course of therapy as we observe how well a particular client responds to each method. Such alterations are necessary. That which instructs, interests and motivates one client may confuse, bore or frustrate another.

Successful R therapy is not for the uninterested, undetermined or unimaginative therapist! It is like the work of a great chef who combines various ingredients in creative ways to devise a brand new recipe every day. Great therapists know the value of various procedures and are willing to adjust them for the specific needs of their clients. Therapists, therefore, are responsible to learn a wide variety of stimulation techniques so that the most effective ones can be selected. They also must be able to change their minds about techniques at a moments notice so that procedures can fit the immediate needs of clients. These things are true for all aspects of speech and language therapy, and they are especially true for remediation of R.

Stimulation Techniques

Stimulation techniques pique the senses so that appropriate speech movements occur and the sound of R results. Stimulation techniques for articulation therapy are auditory, visual, tactile and proprioceptive in nature.

- *Auditory stimulation* is used to help clients hear R as a distinct unit of sound and to discriminate fine differences in its production. Auditory discrimination helps clients monitor the sound while making oral-position changes. It is the most important element of articulation therapy. Without the ability to hear, an R is almost impossible to learn.
- *Visual stimulation* is used to help clients understand how the jaw, lips and tongue move in and out of position for R. Clients try to match their own oral movements to the given visual image. Visual feedback helps them monitor their movements. Visual information helps the learning process, but it is not critical. After all, most children naturally learn R without ever studying their mouths in a mirror. Even a person with no sight can learn the sound.
- *Tactile stimulation* is used to facilitate specific oral movements for the production of R. Tactile stimulation also is used to normalize oral-tactile sensitivity so that clients can perceive fine movement changes in the mouth based on tactile feedback. Tactile feedback helps clients perceive their own oral movements, positions and tension.
- *Proprioceptive stimulation* is used to normalize muscular tone so the jaw, lips and tongue can move successfully for R production. Proprioceptive stimulation also

is used to facilitate specific movements for the production of R. Proprioceptive feedback ultimately is that which informs clients about their own oral positions.

Real Kids

The following are real cases that bridge the gap between assessment and treatment. As stated earlier, it is quite tempting to limit our discussion in this book to clients who have R as their only speech problem. However, the reality of daily therapy is that clients with problematic R usually have other issues too. Each case study includes a brief summary of background information, treatment procedures and results of therapy. All names have been changed to protect privacy, except for my daughter Namasté, who wanted her real name to be used.

Martin: A Surprise R with Severe Dysarthria

BACKGROUND

Martin came to me at four years of age with severe dysarthria caused by muscular dystrophy. He used about 25 words that he said with only one vowel and two consonants. He was almost completely unintelligible, unless you already knew what he was talking about. Martin demonstrated severe oral-motor disorder with very limited oral movement, hypersensitivity, and excessive drooling. Cognitive and expressive language was delayed. At age four, Martin functioned like a 24-month-old.

TREATMENT

Our language work centered on building concepts, expressive vocabulary and early word combinations. Oral-motor therapy was used to normalize oral-tactile sensitivity and to improve oral awareness and basic control of the jaw, lips and tongue. It included feeding techniques and oral-exploratory play with a wide variety of oral toys and tools. In articulation, we worked intensively on the vowels and prosodic features of speech to boost intelligibility. We worked on all the stop consonants as well as some of the nasals and glides. I did not target R specifically, because of the severity of his speech and language disorder. I figured it would be many years before Martin would be able to say an R—if ever.

RESULTS

Two years later, Martin's expressive speech had reached the four-to-five word utterance level and he used a wide variety of vowels and consonants. He was about 60 percent intelligible with known and familiar topics but still very difficult to understand with unknown ones. Oral skills had improved significantly. However, drooling was still a severe problem and was managed with medication. Out of the blue, and without ever really focusing on the sound, R made an appearance on the word *car*. Martin said *car* with a beautiful Tip R at the end of the word but with no consonant at the beginning of the word. Noticing the new R, I targeted it on and off for several months in the final position intermixed with his other work. We worked on rhyming words *bar, far, jar, star* and then two-syllable words, like *soccer, player, jumper* and others. I was able to establish R in the final position of all words. One year later, Martin was using utterances of eight and more words in length. The R remained solid in the final position. We were not so fortunate with more basic consonants like W, K and G. And R had not generalized to the initial position.

LESSONS LEARNED
- Don't exclude R from your training with clients who demonstrate severe speech disorder or who are enrolled for other reasons. Correct R may not be a specific goal of treatment, but techniques to facilitate its emergence can be included under the umbrella of facilitating general articulation and phonological development. This is true even in cases of severe dysarthria or apraxia.
- R is not always the last sound to emerge. It can come in early.
- R does not always emerge in the initial position. The final, or post-vocalic, position often is the place R makes its first appearance.

John: Success with the Nasal Substitute

BACKGROUND

John came to me at eleven years of age with a non-English, voiceless substitute for R. It was a soft nasal puff of sound. (Think about that for a minute.) He was bright and talkative, yet somewhat difficult to understand because of the R misarticulation and its hypernasal effect on other nearby consonants and vowels.

TREATMENT

John was enrolled in weekly half-hour sessions. Our first goal was to establish an oral sound for R, no matter how distorted that sound was. Our second goal was to shape this oral sound into R using ear training and oral-motor techniques. We worked on the Tip R. Some focus was put on L because it was produced with inconsistent tongue-tip placement and was distorted intermittently. We built from L to R using both the slide and tapping procedures.

RESULTS

John established an oral sound within a few months of treatment. The tool that was the most effective in teaching him to become oral while attempting R was a 12-inch piece of vinyl tubing. One end was placed at his nose or mouth and the other at his ear while he practiced some of the vowels and the nasals M, N, and Ng. This taught him to recognize when sound came out his nose verses his mouth. Once he was able to discriminate consistently, we were able to transfer this skill to his productions of R. He also placed his finger on his nose to feel the nasal vibration on R while he used the tube at his ear. Weeks later, we stopped using the tube. John was able to identify nasal vibration consistently with his finger. Finally, he was able to stop using his finger to monitor the nasality. He could feel it in his nose, and his ear began to pick up the error.

Once John learned to make a consistent oral sound, we turned our attention to correct oral position for R. Learning the correct jaw and tongue movements to use with the new oral sound proved difficult, but he learned them in a few months. When an acoustically correct R began to emerge, it showed up first in the final position of simple words like *far, jar* and *star*. Once these words stabilized, we were able to isolate the sound and eventually transfer it to the initial position of words.

Seven months into treatment, John was rehearsing a wide variety of words with R in all positions. We switched to telephone therapy. I called him once a week for fifteen minutes. He lived quite far away. Phone therapy allowed us to continue rehearsal over the next two months without the added time needed to travel to my office. During this time, I also saw him in my office twice to check the sound in the live acoustic space.

As of this writing, John has taken the summer off from therapy. I will check him again soon. Depending upon his performance, I will take one of three courses of action. If he has maintained his skill, I will discontinue his service or I will continue to follow-up for a few more months. If he has slipped into old habits, I will initiate weekly therapy again to bring him up to prior performance levels, and then repeat the tapering-off process.

LESSONS LEARNED
- Don't treat a nasal substitute lightly. Target the oral-nasal problem first and make sure to establish the oral sound no matter how distorted it is. Treat the oral-movement problem second.
- Be flexible in treatment scheduling. Even something as radical as telephone therapy can be effective for some clients.
- Don't worry about time off from therapy. It can be a necessary break to see how effective the work has been.

Theresa: Quitting in the Face of Refusal and an Incomplete Diagnosis

BACKGROUND
I consider Theresa to be my worst failure in R therapy. She came to me at the age of eleven for a severe R distortion. However, her speech was characterized by other features: very rapid rate, monotone, periodic hypernasality, inconsistent omission of sounds and syllables, a muffled quality and a high level of unintelligibility. Theresa, however, was oblivious to the fact that people had difficulty understanding her. She chattered away incessantly despite frequent requests for clarification. The listener eventually got the gist of her message if he listened long enough. Theresa was completely uninterested in whether anyone understood her. She left almost no room for anyone else to speak. Theresa talked mostly on certain topics, and she was very rigid in most of her activities and routines. Theresa read with exceptional skill at least four years above age level equivalency.

TREATMENT
We began weekly thirty-minute sessions to address R as well as rate, intonation and articulatory precision. Theresa rejected all the work I presented except for practice on R. She insisted that R was the only reason that she came to therapy, stating clearly on

numerous occasions that she did not find anything wrong with her R. She came to therapy only because her parents insisted.

As one might imagine, I got nowhere with this child. For four months she refused to work on rate or rhythm. She would not imitate any specific oral movements, finding them "very gross." She never pronounced one R sound correctly. However, at home Theresa was merrily making lists of R words and practicing them in front of the bathroom mirror. She rehearsed with lots of flourish and drama but with no correct R sounds. In essence, Theresa ignored everything I asked her to do, and designed her own treatment program organized around rehearsing distorted R's. What a whirlwind she was!

RESULTS

Theresa was dismissed from therapy after four months with absolutely no change. Her parents and I were frustrated, but there was nothing we could do to get through to her. She spoke of becoming a famous actress who would one day be known for her interesting speech patterns. She wanted to keep everything just the way it was. Despite my dismay, I had to admire her persistent drive to be herself. I thought she was just a stubborn preadolescent acting out her life's fantasy. Thinking back on her behavior, I am convinced Theresa had mild undiagnosed Autism or Asperger's Syndrome. But no such idea entered my mind then. I designed my treatment for her as if she were a normal rebellious child with a complicated expressive speech problem.

LESSONS LEARNED

- You can lead a horse to water, but you can't make him drink.
- Understanding the etiology of a misarticulated R is critical to a successful outcome. Without it you are the blind leading the blind.
- Children with other syndromes can have misarticulation of R and other phonemes. These children must be handled differently than the average child. Programming must be designed to fit into their personal learning and communication style.
- Failure in R therapy should not deter us from taking on the next case. Each case, be it completed with success or failure, should be viewed as a learning experience to hone professional skills.

Jasmine: Easy Success with the Dream Client

BACKGROUND

Jasmine came to me at seven years of age with an R distortion and no other expressive speech or language problems. She was bright, talkative and interested in attending therapy. She was trying to make a Back R by lifting the middle back of her tongue instead of the lateral backs, and she was positioning her lips so that a V sound was added to it. She also did not have enough tension in the tongue to get the right acoustic quality. When asked why she had come to therapy, she said, "Because I want to learn my R." Yes!

TREATMENT

Jasmine and I engaged in weekly thirty-minute sessions that focused on getting the tongue in the right position and tensing it correctly for the Back R. We used a few simple oral-motor procedures and auditory discrimination work. Most of our activities involved drawing. She loved colored markers and the freedom to create her own pictures.

RESULTS

Jasmine learned to say R correctly and consistently within two months. She continued in weekly therapy for another three months to establish the sound in all positions and in conversation. She was recalled for follow-up three months after dismissal and was scheduled for two brush-up sessions to complete correct use of R in a few phonetic environments. She was rechecked again three months later and had maintained full control. Six months later I called the mother again to see if my services were needed anymore. The mom said, "Hey, I think we're done!" I agreed.

LESSONS LEARNED

- There are dream clients who understand the problem, who enthusiastically comply with treatment procedures, and who fix up their problem in no time.
- Despite the ease with which some clients learn R, the overall treatment process can take at least one year.

Steve and Patty: The Simple Boost

BACKGROUND

Steve came to me at the age of five with a distorted R and no other developmental issues or speech/language problems. He was the middle child of three. His older sister had no speech errors.

TREATMENT

I saw Steve for an initial evaluation and was able to stimulate a wonderful postvocalic Tip R almost immediately. We rehearsed this sound for ten minutes, then went on to words. Immediately, Steve said words containing final R with near perfect mastery. The parents and I decided that I would see him again in a few months to determine if a boost was all he would need.

RESULTS

When I saw Steve again, he was using a correct R about 95 percent of the time in rapid conversational speech and he was self-correcting on the few words that tripped him up. We rehearsed many tricky words. We decided to have one more follow-up session five months later. When I called to set up this appointment, the mother said he was doing great and needed no further help. She still wanted to come in, however, but this time to bring the younger sister who had the same error! I saw Patty when she was only four years old. She also learned R in the first session and followed the same course of improvement.

LESSONS LEARNED
- A simple boost is all that is needed in some cases. When this is seen, periodic follow-up sessions once every few months should be scheduled to monitor progress. Follow-up sessions help ensure that the client does not fail to acquire R in rare or complicated words.
- The misarticulated R can be noted in several members of a single family. No scientific studies have identified a cause of familial patterns. Sometimes a child's error can be due to simple imitation of error sounds modeled by adults or older siblings.
- Clients who demonstrate an error on R and no other phonemes, and who learn R with a simple boost, have perfectly intact auditory discrimination and oral-motor skills. They simply have not learned how to say R. Once they learn it, they can transfer this skill almost immediately to all phonetic contexts.
- In the public school, three boost sessions during the schoolyear can be an excellent way to ensure that those students who should be able to grow out of an R error actually do. Consider scheduling one day of boost sessions per trimester. Use that whole day (or half day) to see all these clients one after another. Clients who do not benefit from scheduled boost sessions should be enrolled in weekly treatment.

Eileen: Singing Tips for Vocal Projection

BACKGROUND

Eileen came to me as a sixth-grade student with good grades and a singing background. She was enrolled in a private girls' choir and was quite good as a soprano. I had heard her sing many times because one of my daughters also was in this choir. Distorted R was Eileen's only error phoneme. She had made some incomplete progress in her school-based articulation program. She was referred to me for outside help to conquer the error before she went on to junior high. Needless to say, I was nervous in taking this case. I have a policy never to treat my friends' children. Although I did not know this family at the time, our lives overlapped at school, choir, in the neighborhood and at the elementary school. I knew I could not fail here, and I had reservations because R therapy can be so problematic.

TREATMENT

I was doing home-based treatment at the time and scheduled Eileen for one thirty-minute session per week. We worked at her kitchen table when other family members were away and it was quiet. Eileen was producing a sound almost like R when we began. With a little work on tongue control and oral position, she was able to attain a decent R position in two sessions. What was really holding Eileen back was that her R sounded muffled, like it was stuck in the back of her throat. I ignored this for several weeks, assuming that the problem would go away and a clear R would emerge. It didn't. I had to think of a way to get this sound out. I began asking Eileen to sit up straight and speak louder. That helped a little, but it didn't remediate the problem.

Then I thought about how she worked with her voice when she sang. Her vocal instructor got the children to project their voices. I adopted the same terminology and worked with simple vowels. I asked her to prolong these sounds and to project her voice while saying them. I told her to "make the sounds come all the way out like you do when you sing." I used my arms to demonstrate the movement of sound from inside the mouth to a point a full arm's length away from the mouth. Eileen already knew how to project voice to make a chest voice and a head voice, so we equated these ideas with our work on the vowels and then on R. I said, "Make the sound stand out in front of you," and, "Sing the sound so it moves out and away from you."

RESULTS

She did it! Her production of R became perfect almost immediately. Once Eileen had the idea of projecting her voice appropriately, it took only a few weeks for her to take hold of this skill at all levels of training, from isolated R productions to conversational speech. She finished the treatment process in about four months. Eileen is in college now, and I am happy to report that she maintained her R and is studying opera. During her senior recital at the end of high school, she accredited some of her vocal success to the R therapy she received in elementary school!

LESSONS LEARNED

- Therapy can be highly successful when key elements of treatment are identified and addressed. Failure may be inevitable when underlying factors are ignored or overlooked. These things are true in all levels of articulation therapy, from severe dysarthria and apraxia to the "simple" misarticulated R.
- Oral position is not enough when learning R. The ability to produce and project good voice is integral to successful R therapy.
- Speech and language pathologists can acquire much needed information about voice for R and other phonemes from the study of vocal training for singing. Many of the ideas overlap, and the terms are useful.
- A quiet environment with few distractions is necessary for good articulation therapy. Even old-fashioned "kitchen-table therapy" can be successful under these conditions. Articulation therapy in the classroom is not recommended for R therapy and other types of articulation and phonological therapies, because there are many uncontrolled auditory and visual distractions.
- A well-produced R can be a necessary and critical component of reaching lifetime goals.

Ben: Postponing Therapy until the Time Is Right

BACKGROUND

Ben came to me at the age of eleven with a classic R distortion and an otherwise intact speech production system. He did not want to attend therapy. "My friends don't notice anything. I don't see why it's a problem." Ben would have have come to therapy if his parents had insisted, but he had no interest. Ben was a little antagonistic, and adolescence rebellion was lurking around the corner. I was afraid that we would lose him for good if we pushed. Reevaluation was scheduled for the following spring. Upon recall one year later, when he was twelve, Ben was singing a new tune. Someone in his school had made fun of his R that year, and he was now committed and ready to begin therapy.

TREATMENT

Therapy was scheduled for weekly thirty-minute sessions. It included standard procedures for establishing a Tip R, including auditory discrimination and basic instruction on oral position.

RESULTS

Ben learned R easily and finished the process in five months. Follow-up lasted for another six months.

LESSONS LEARNED

- It is better to postpone R therapy until the child is ready, than to insist on it when he's not committed.
- Peer pressure can have an enormous influence on a young client's perception of the R problem and his willingness to participate in its remediation.

Namasté: R Therapy for Toddlers

BACKGROUND

My youngest daughter, Namasté (pronounced *NAH-mah-stay*), was slow to talk. Her first words did not appear until 17 months. Thankfully, expressive speech and language developed quickly after that. She caught up at 24 months of age. However, much to my horror, she arrived at age two-and-a-half with a distorted R. All of my professional friends, of course, assured me there was nothing to worry about. After all, she was only two years of age. But I knew R's. This was not a developmental error. This was a true R distortion, the kind that never goes away without treatment. I decided to wait one year before intervening. Six months later, at her third birthday, Namasté's distorted R was fixed in position. She was making a Back R with high elevation of the tongue's middle-back section—the worst error of all. Further, her two older sisters were beginning to mock her R production by imitating this sound. This distorted R was everywhere in my home. I decided that I had to do something about it or my professional life was over.

TREATMENT

Two-year-olds are not known for their compliant behavior, and Namasté was no exception. I had to design activities that would help her learn sound without her knowing that we were doing anything out of the ordinary. I began daily play-therapy with Namasté. I determined that once a day when she and I had a few moments alone, I would engage in her favorite types of gross motor play, including tickling, hugging, spinning, swinging, bouncing, tumbling around, and so forth. While engaged in these playful interchanges, I incorporated four types of treatment activities.

1. We "played" with all the vowels and the voiced consonants by incorporating them into our physical play. For example, we chanted "oo-oo-oo-oo" while she bounced on my lap.
2. We opened our mouths wide to "play" with our tongues. We stretched our tongue tips to all parts of the mouth, from extending far outside the mouth to curling it far back into the deep recesses of the oral cavity like a Tip R. This was done while working face-to-face.
3. We babbled silly words that began with the glides W, L, Y and R. For example, we played with "Ah-Yah-Yah" and "Oh-Woh-Woh." The R sound in these sequences was made with a grand sweep up and back with the tongue tip. These productions did two things: They helped her differentiate all four glides one from another, and they helped her learn to say a Tip R.
4. I modeled a W-for-R substitution in real words. This I could do at any time of the day. We said "wain" for *rain* and "wabbit" for *rabbit*. This was to break her habit of using the distorted R and to train her to use the more normal substitution. My older girls helped out with this. They especially liked saying "Mr. Wogers" for their television idol.

RESULTS

Daily treatment sessions faded to weekly and then monthly. Namasté completed the entire process in less than one year. No sign of an R distortion was present by her fourth birthday. Now, there is no way that I can prove she would not have done this on her own. But I am certain that she would not have. She had learned an incorrect oral-motor pattern for R, the precise one that plagues many speech and language pathologists as the "unfixable" R. It was clear that this sound was becoming locked in, and that remediation would eventually be needed. We could have done it later, but with my work specializing in the treatment of R and other articulation problems, I simply *had* to do it early. Also, I had to see if it *could* be done early. I was pleased and quite relieved to see that it could.

LESSONS LEARNED

- Certain R distortions are not developmental in nature, especially the distorted R made with a high middle back.
- Therapy for the distorted R can be addressed during the toddler and preschool years by engaging in playful activities. Early intervention prevents the distorted R from locking in for a lifetime.
- A toddler with an isolated incorrect R would not likely be enrolled in articulation therapy, but he could be. Treatment can take a playful approach.

Davie: Family Problems Interfere with Treatment

BACKGROUND

Davie came to me at four years of age with a number of minor phoneme errors, including a simple W-for-R substitution. I assured the parents that at his age, these errors could wait but that I would be glad to help him now if they were interested. During the initial examination, I discovered that the parents were separated and in the middle of a divorce. Right in front of me they blamed each other for the problems they had, including Davie's minor speech delay. They argued about the need for treatment. She wanted him to get it now; he wanted to wait. They even haggled about who would pay for the day's evaluation. The session ended with no plan. I asked the parents to talk this over. I promised to call in one week to see if they had decided to set up a therapy schedule. I knew that this family had much bigger issues to worry about.

TREATMENT
Subsequent telephone messages left at the home were never returned. Treatment was never initiated.

RESULTS
Unknown.

LESSONS LEARNED
- Family problems can interfere with the treatment process of private practice. The home must be cooperative in getting the child to treatment, in paying the bill, and in engaging in some home practice. A child and his family have to be ready for the weekly commitment to the process.
- Public-school speech and language pathologists often are at a disadvantage in this regard. School therapists usually do not know much about the home situation and typically must enroll students in therapy despite it. Some clients fail in school-based R therapy because their minds are preoccupied with more pressing issues regarding their parents, their friends or their grades.
- Sometimes our hearts break when we know we can help a child but circumstances prevent us from being able to do so.

Arnold: Frontal Lisp, Lateral Lisp, Distorted R, Hypersensitivity

BACKGROUND
Arnold came to me as a five-year-old boy in preschool with a distorted R, a frontal lisp on S and Z, and a lateral lisp on the palatal sibilants. In addition, Arnold dropped many final consonants, had no L, and reduced clusters to single sounds. He was approximately 25 percent unintelligible in rapid conversational speech. Arnold's attention, oculomotor and oral-motor skills were quite poor, and the parents were holding him back from kindergarten until the next year.

TREATMENT
Arnold was enrolled in therapy for almost one year. During that time, we worked on a wide variety of speech sounds and phonological processes. He closed syllables, gained L, and began to use all the clusters. Intelligibility improved considerably. With only the frontal lisp,

lateral lisp and distorted R left, we dismissed him from private therapy when he entered kindergarten. I was concerned that he did not qualify for school therapy. However, his mother wanted to see if he could fix the rest of his problems on his own. Arnold returned to me the following summer at age six with no change. He still had the frontal lisp, lateral lisp and distorted R. That summer, we worked on developing a consistent midline sibilant sound and a Tip R with extensive oral-motor procedures.

RESULTS

As of this writing, Arnold is still on my caseload and has just been dismissed for another break. He has received a full year of continuous treatment this time, and he has almost completely conquered his R. We are taking a break because of this success on R. His sibilants are still problematic, however, because he is in the process of losing deciduous teeth and cannot count on the correct sound of the sibilants for more than a few weeks at a time. Over time, it has become increasingly clear to me that Arnold's oral hypersensitivity has been a significant factor in phoneme learning. He used to gag when attempting a Tip R or when touching even the anterior parts of his mouth. This is resolving with time and specific oral-motor work, which is allowing him to produce R consistently. I will monitor Arnold's speech every three months during this schoolyear to make sure the R stays on track, and we will probably do weekly therapy next summer to address the sibilants again.

LESSONS LEARNED

- Children with the threefold problem of frontal lisp, lateral lisp and distorted R should not be excluded from therapy in the early years. This constellation of errors strongly suggests a deeper problem and a more urgent need for remediation. This is especially true if even more errors existed earlier in the child's development.
- A combination of frontal lisp, lateral lisp and distorted R and L is a direct sign of an oral-motor deficit. These are not speech errors, *per se*. These are oral-movement errors. In essence, the client is moving the mouth in incorrect patterns and he is using these aberrant patterns to produce speech sounds. The sibilants and other advanced sounds, like R and L, are the most effected.
- Oral-tactile hypersensitivity can have a devastating effect on articulation skill, even in mild to moderate cases. Hypersensitivity forces a client to avoid the very oral movements that can help them learn to make correct sounds. Articulation therapy improves significantly when sensitivity is normalized.

Melody: Thumbsucking, Occlusion Problems and R Distortion

BACKGROUND

At eight years of age, Melody had a classic combination of problems: frontal lisp, distorted L and R, anterior open bite, reverse swallow pattern, open-lips resting posture, and a strong thumbsucking habit. She had learned not to suck while out in public, but it was a strong habit at home during the day, at night and in the car.

TREATMENT

It was determined that the thumbsucking habit was the culprit behind all the other problems. The thumbsucking habit caused the severe anterior open bite, and it perpetuated the reverse swallow pattern and open-lips rest posture. The reverse swallow pattern prevented development of good tongue bowling with tip- and lateral-margin elevation. The tongue had learned to work incorrectly with high elevation of the midline and lack of elevation of the tip and sides. Distortion of L, R and the sibilants were the result.

Melody was referred to a speech and language pathologist who specialized in the elimination of oral habits. During that schoolyear, when she was ready and with the help of the therapist, Melody eliminated her thumbsucking habit. Once the oral habit was gone, the therapist taught her correct tongue position during oral rest. Then she received upper and lower braces to help pull the teeth back into correct alignment. Six months into orthodontia, Melody received a few lessons on correct swallowing. Six months after that, her speech was checked again, and she received a few lessons on correct tongue movement for L and the sibilants.

RESULTS

Melody never did receive direct work on R, yet it emerged on its own after she had been helped to attain the best structural and functional environment for it.

LESSONS LEARNED

- An oral habit like thumbsucking can cause the development of incorrect oral movements, swallow pattern and oral-rest posture. Distortion of R and other phonemes can result.
- Elimination of an oral habit sets the stage for correct oral function to emerge. It is the combination of treatment for oral structure, oral habits, oral-rest position and swallowing that makes for a successful program. Sometimes R and other phonemes straighten themselves out with little or no direct intervention after the structural and habitual changes.
- In most cases, malocclusion by itself should *not* interfere with the emergence of R. The teeth do not have to be perfectly aligned for R to emerge. However, malocclusion can be an indication of incorrect oral function. It is the presence of improper oral movement that can preclude R and other phonemes from emerging.

Looking Ahead to Therapy

These case studies have been provided to help readers gain a broad overview of the process of articulation therapy for the misarticulated R phoneme. They have demonstrated that R therapy is not always simple, nor is it always successful. The rest of this book is devoted to the successful side of this story. The therapy material is organized by type of stimulation and benefit of technique. As such, each chapter tackles one avenue of successful treatment.

~ Summary ~

- Therapy can be interesting and amusing for both client and instructor. Scientific facts must be translated into everyday language to fit the imaginations of our clients.

- There is no right or wrong techniques in R therapy. Every technique is valuable, no matter its genre. The therapist's job is to find the right solution for each and every client. Therapy is like the work of a great chef who puts various ingredients together in creative ways to invent new recipes.

- Stimulation techniques pique the senses so that appropriate speech movements occur. They are auditory, visual, tactile and proprioceptive in nature.

- R therapy is appropriate for clients with severe dysarthria or apraxia. The initiation of R therapy for these clients is determined by the individual client's readiness for such treatment.

- R may emerge early and in the final position of words before other developmentally appropriate phonemes and phonological patterns emerge.

- Nasality problems and oral-movement problems related to R are addressed in that order.

- Flexibility in treatment scheduling is important. Don't worry about time off from therapy, and feel free to postpone it until the child is ready.

- Peer pressure has a huge influence on a young person's perception of the R problem and his willingness to participate in its remediation.

- R therapy can fail when other pervasive learning problems are present.

- Unlike the W-for-R substitution, the distorted R is not a developmental pattern that goes away easily.

- R therapy can be done with toddlers in playful ways. Early treatment prevents an incorrect R pattern from locking in for a lifetime.

- Family problems can interfere with the treatment process. Sometimes our hearts break when we know we can help children but circumstances prevent us from being able to do so.

- Children with R distortion, frontal lisp and lateral lisp should not be excluded from early therapy. This constellation of behaviors strongly suggests an oral-motor basis and a need for immediate remediation.

- Oral-tactile hypersensitivity can have a devastating effect on R learning because it can prevent specific oral-movement patterns from emerging.

- An oral habit like thumbsucking can cause incorrect oral movements to develop. Incorrect swallow and oral rest as well as distortion of R and other phonemes can result.

- Malocclusion should *not* interfere with the emergence of R in most cases. However, malocclusion is an indication of incorrect oral movement, and it is that improper oral movement that may preclude R and other phonemes from emerging.

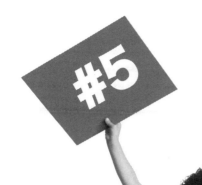

Listening and Learning
The Essential Work of Auditory Stimulation

Despite the popularity and necessity of oral-motor therapy in today's speech and language clinic, auditory skill training remains the primary tool of articulation therapy. It is the most important of all the sensory stimulation channels in sound acquisition because we must be able to hear phonemes before we can really understand how to produce them. That is why we begin our discussion of R therapy here. Auditory stimulation trains a client to recognize R as a unique sound and to differentiate a correct R from its deviations. Auditory stimulation is perhaps the easiest and most widely used method of all the stimulation techniques available. It is the least invasive, requires the fewest pieces of equipment, and is the most efficient to use in group therapy. Further, auditory discrimination will teach your client how to achieve and monitor correct oral position for production of the sound.

The best programs of articulation therapy include methods for stimulating both auditory and oral-motor skills. These two approaches can be combined together in three ways throughout the course of treatment for the misarticulated R. We can:

1. Begin therapy with auditory work and initiate oral-motor work later.
2. Integrate auditory and oral-motor work together from the beginning.
3. Begin with oral-motor work and initiate auditory work later.

There are advantages and drawbacks to each approach as described in the next three sections.

Auditory Work First
Most articulation programs begin with auditory work. This is because so many children can learn R from auditory stimulation alone. In fact, many children who cannot pronounce R during the preschool years will learn it outside of speech therapy in their kindergarten classrooms during the time in which their teacher instructs them on letter R. The alphabet and pre-reading work done in the typical kindergarten classroom is largely auditory and visual in nature. It can facilitate emergence of R in many children. These children have intact oral-motor skills and can learn R from the cursory auditory and visual training

done in the classroom. Children who cannot learn R from classroom training may require some individual or small-group articulation therapy. For them, we do auditory work first to prevent us from wasting time in other areas. Auditory work helps clients define correct and incorrect R sounds with the ear. Some clients will begin to produce better R sounds as a result of this simple introduction—the easiest of the easy clients. If auditory work alone does not cause R to emerge, other work, described in subsequent chapters, must be added.

Simultaneous Auditory and Oral-Motor Work
There are always a significant number of clients who cannot learn R from auditory work alone, either in the classroom or in speech therapy. In these cases, auditory training is provided simultaneously with oral-motor training from the beginning so that the two areas complement each other. Such coordinated training always is necessary when deficits in oral-motor development are present. The balance of the program's sessions will include some auditory training and some oral-motor work. The time spent on each area may be divided in half in each session, or the two areas may be integrated by switching from one to the other every few minutes within the session. Some sessions will focus entirely on one area or the other. These decisions are at the discretion of the speech and language pathologist, and they depend upon the client's immediate responses to techniques.

It is safe to say that most clients with longterm misarticulation of R fit this category. They need both auditory and oral-motor work throughout their program. In fact, many clients who are failing in longterm R therapy are doing so because the work is leaning too heavily in one direction or the other. In past decades, this usually meant that auditory training was the only stimulation being used. Today, unfortunately, the opposite is true. Clients are failing in R therapy because too much focus is put on oral-motor work. A balanced approach to R therapy that includes both auditory and oral-motor work is necessary for the bulk of our clients. This is true even if the auditory work consists only of an instruction to listen, and the oral-motor work simply includes the command, "Do this . . ."

Ultimately our clients need to be taught how to listen carefully to their own sound productions while they alter jaw, lip and tongue positions slightly. This is the integration of auditory and oral-motor work that an infant naturally uses to learn all of his sounds. When the listening system and the oral-movement system work together, a client can discover, practice and conquer his distorted R.

Oral-Motor Work First
It may be a shock to some readers to realize that there are significant numbers of clients who cannot discriminate the correct acoustic quality of an R sound until *after* they have learned to produce it correctly. In other words, they learn to hear R by saying it. This may seem backward, but it mirrors the way little babies learn to produce sound. Babies do not set out to learn a B, a W, an M or even an R. Instead, they produce a wide variety of sounds spontaneously and learn to recognize and take control of these sounds through playful experimentation. In other words, the mouth teaches the ear to hear. Clients who learn to hear R only after they can speak it are learning R in the natural way that most young

children do. They simply cannot hear R until after they have spent time producing a correct one.

Experienced therapists recognize these clients. They are the ones who produce one or two R's correctly each session but always return the next session as if they had learned nothing the time before. They also are the ones who seem completely unimpressed when we tell them, "That was a great one!" Our enthusiasm means nothing to them because they cannot hear it. To them, the great sound they just produced is no more impressive than the hundreds they produced poorly. These clients must be taught to make the correct R sound even though they cannot hear it. We do this by facilitating and rehearsing oral position. When the client chances upon a correct sound, we tell him, "That's it!" We do not ask him what he thought about his production, because he does not know. Instead we tell him, "That's the one we want." These clients are highly dependent upon their therapists to tell them what is correct and incorrect in each of their productions early in therapy.

Auditory Stimulation

Auditory stimulation takes several different forms that work together to help clients develop the ability to recognize and discriminate the R sound by listening to it. The techniques suggested in the rest of this chapter cover all aspects of auditory training. Some of the oldest methods are presented first. After that, the techniques are organized in no special sequence. All auditory training exercises are based around the client listening to sounds produced by others and by himself.

The *auditory cue* is the sound of R as it is produced by the attending therapist. Therapists produce R models so that clients can listen to them and engage in listening training. At the center of R therapy is a correct vocal model provided by the therapist to the client. This auditory cue is the seed of virtually the entire remediation program. It is imperative, therefore, that the practicing speech and language pathologist be able to produce a correct R sound in all positions of words, and that she can do so automatically and consistently in rapid conversational speech. Therapists who cannot produce correct R sounds are ethically bound to refer their clients with R misarticulation to another speech and language pathologist who can.

The activities in this chapter and the rest of this book assume a normal range of hearing acuity on the part of the client. Adaptations must be made if hearing acuity is outside normal range.

Basic Auditory Attention

Auditory attention refers simply to the client's ability to actively listen to a target sound. In R therapy, auditory attention is designed to pull the client's attention away from other things and to draw it to the sound of R as a unique phonetic unit. Auditory attention training often begins with gross listening, and progresses to fine-listening activities.

GROSS-LISTENING ACTIVITIES

With younger children, the first few sessions of R therapy often begin with warm-up activities to get the client to pay attention to general sound. This can be done in hundreds of different ways. For example, place five common items on a table—a stapler, a box of paper clips, a pen with a clicking mechanism, a pair of scissors and a pad of paper. Make a noise with one of the objects while the child's eyes are closed or the objects are hidden behind a screen. For example, snip the air with the scissors, or flip through the pad of paper. Then ask the client to guess which item was used. Reverse rolls and alternate turns. This activity will help the client focus his auditory attention on gross sounds. Any items that make sound will do for this activity, including common objects or musical instruments.

As another simple example, ask your client to sit very still and listen for sound in the environment. What does he hear? He might hear a clanging radiator, a buzzing light fixture, a child talking in the hall, a ticking clock, traffic rushing by, the siren of an ambulance in the distance, a telephone ringing, or rain beating on the window. Such an activity will get kids to settle down and open their ears to subtle sounds. Listen carefully. Then ask the client to plug his ears with his fingers. Can he hear all of the sounds now?

Another idea to stimulate gross auditory attention is to use a radio with a dial tuner. Start with the dial position all the way to the left of the dial. Ask the client to turn the dial slowly to the right in order to sweep the stations. Ask him to stop when he hears a station coming in, and then teach him how to tune it in well. Some kids will already know how to do this. Still, it is an excellent and fun activity. Remember, the purpose of gross auditory stimulation is to train the client to pay attention to gross sounds in active ways.

RHYMING WORDS

It has been my experience that many clients in articulation therapy do not understand rhyming words. They have not gone through that developmental stage in which children find rhyming to be fun and funny. Often, this is a reflection of their poorly developed auditory discrimination skills. Auditory skills can be enhanced when we teach our clients the beauty of words that rhyme. This can be done with nursery rhymes, songs or poems. Dr. Seuss books are perfect for working on rhyming words. Spend some time listening to and producing rhymes to facilitate auditory awareness and discrimination of speech sound. Do this as an aside to treatment, as a break away from the more difficult work they may need. It will seem like a break to the child, but it is excellent auditory attention training.

WORDPLAY

Another way to get clients to listen carefully to gross word productions is to play with words. For young children, this often means playing with *wrong* words. A wrong-word activity entails saying a wrong word purposefully in order to have fun while listening hard. For example, sing a child's song and substitute an incorrect word at a certain point each time you sing the refrain. In "Mary Had a Little Lamb," substitute a different animal name in place of the word *lamb*. Make it sillier by using non-animal words, like, "Mary had a little shoe, little shoe, little shoe. . . ." Young children love these silly wordplay activities. They help them listen hard and tune their ears to the words of others.

ADVANCED WORDPLAY

Wordplay can be done with older children to enhance listening skills, but it must be more subtle than the wrong-word training. At this level, we move into an investigation of words themselves. For example, one day a fourteen-year-old R client of mine became fascinated with the word *phoneme*, a word that she noticed I had written in the notes I was making during her session. She asked what it meant, and we discussed it. We dug into the meanings of the words *telephone, microphone, megaphone, phonetics* and *phonology*. She noted the similarity between the base words, *phon* and *photo,* so we branched into a discussion of the base word *photo* and discussed *photograph, photography* and *photosynthesis.*

To a casual observer, it may have seemed as if the girl and I were avoiding our work on R for fifteen minutes. To the contrary! This type of word comparison enhances an older client's auditory discrimination skills in a way that also piques curiosity and interest. One is motivated to listen hard to words that contain similar roots. There is no better way to help a client listen to speech. The older child's reaction to this work is one of interest and curiosity, rather than fun and silliness, as seen in younger clients working on rhyming words. The child is engaged in the listening process and developing auditory attention skills. By the way, I have worked with many older children who could not rhyme words. Age is not the factor in gaining these skills; auditory attention and cognitive growth are.

FINE AUDITORY ATTENTION

Auditory attention is refined when we move from environmental sounds and words to the sounds of phonemes. Most children enter speech and language therapy without having thought too much about the idea of speech sounds. They may know the alphabet and may even know how to spell and sound out words, but they may have only a vague notion of the acoustic signal that characterizes R. This is especially true of young children. Refined auditory attention activities are designed to bring the client's focus of attention to the sound of R as it is correctly produced by the therapist. For example, we might say to the client, "What are we here to work on? That's right—R. What does it sound like?" Suddenly the client's focus on other things stops and he is drawn to the idea of the sound of R. He turns his mind and his ear to this topic. Then we might say, "Listen to me. I will say the sound of the letter R. Listen to what it sounds like."

A general discussion about letter R might ensue, with discoveries about the prominence of R in the child's life. Perhaps there is an R in the child's name, or in the name of one or more of his family members or friends. Perhaps his dog's name or the name of his town begins with R. Maybe the name of the child's favorite sport or sports figure contains an R. A nice way to organize this discussion is to write down all these important names or words in a list. Say each word carefully as it is identified, and make a big deal about how to spell it, in order to draw the client's attention to R. "How do you spell your dog's name? Let's see, p-r-i-n-c-e. Did you realize that he has an R in his name? There it is, right there." This list helps focus the child's attention on the prominence of R in his life. It also enables you to use these important words in therapy during subsequent weeks of therapy.

Auditory attention activities are not constructed to test the client. We are not trying to see if he can hear or identify the sound of R in these discussions. Instead, we are trying to teach him to listen to the correct pronunciation of R and to think about it as a concept. This is an abstract concept, so we want to make it concrete in several different ways: by writing down its symbol, by talking about it, by spelling with it, and so forth.

Auditory Discrimination

Auditory discrimination refers to the client's ability to differentiate between speech sounds. Basic auditory discrimination work is designed to teach him to listen for the presence of R sounds in words in several different ways. These activities are presented in a sequence of increasing difficulty.

DISCRIMINATION OF THE PRESENCE OF R

Once the therapist is assured that the client knows what letter R is, activities are initiated to help the client listen for the presence or absence of R in words. The therapist might read a list of words, some of which contain R and others that do not. The client's task is to listen to each word as it is spoken slowly and clearly, and to determine if there is an R in it. Published R programs usually contain many pages with these types of activities. For example, a page might depict a number of small line drawings of common objects, such as a *car, bear, shoe, rabbit, carrot, radio, ball, drum, train* and *rooster*. The words of the pictures are not printed. No visual cues are offered. The client is told to listen to the name of each picture as spoken by the therapist and to determine if there is an R in the word. The client then may draw a circle around each picture that contains an R in its name. As a reward, the child can color one or more of the pictures when the page is completed. Therapists pronounce all words with correct articulation during this early stage because we are training him to listen to the correct R sound. We are not trying to fool him. We are training him to listen. As such, we offer him help in making these decisions.

DISCRIMINATION OF SOUND PLACEMENT

Once a client can determine if R is in a word, therapy expands to include exercises to train the client to listen for the placement of R in a word. For example, the client may be asked to determine if R is at the beginning, middle or end of the words *run, carrot* and *car*. The activity trains the client to listen carefully to an entire word and to determine where he hears an R in it. All modeled words contain R and the therapist pronounces each with correct articulation. An activity might be designed to be totally verbal. The therapist might simply say a word, to which the client may shout out, "Beginning!" or, "Middle!" or, "End."

Shouting always livens up an otherwise boring group session. Make it even more fun by substituting other words for the target responses. Have the kids say "Balloon" for "Beginning," "Muddle" for "Middle," and "End Zone" for "End." Such wordplay makes kids listen and think harder about words, and it usually draws them more deeply into this mundane work.

MINIMAL PAIRS TRAINING

The term *minimal pairs training* refers to the use of word pairs that are alike in all sounds except one. In R therapy, one word in the pair contains R and the other does not, but the words are alike in all other ways. Consider the following minimal pair words:

- *boat* and *rote*
- *feet* and *fear*

- *run* and *bun*
- *bran* and *ban*

One word in each pair contains an R and the other does not. Some rhyme; others don't. Minimal pair words are spoken to the client and studied for similarities and differences. It helps to write these words down for comparison. The client might say, "They both start with B, but only this one has an R." This work is very useful to focus the ear on R. It makes clients listen hard throughout words, and to compare and contrast similar words. For some clients this is a difficult activity.

Differentiation of the Four Glides

One of the most important aspects of auditory discrimination work for stimulation of R entails listening activities to differentiate the four glides W, L, Y and R. These four phonemes are made similarly, and their auditory quality is comparable. That is one of the reasons they are classified together as glides. In normal development, children learn to differentiate this group from all other consonants and vowels, and then they learn to differentiate the four sounds in the group one from another. This second skill has not been achieved by many R clients. The problem manifests as substitution of these sounds one for another. Therefore, activities to help clients differentiate R from W, L and Y are in order.

The easiest way to do this work is to include activities involving all four sounds within the same activity. With young children, consider developing four different characters who say only certain things. For example:

- The first can be a character who cries all the time. He says, "Wah-wah!"
- The second can be a character who sings all the time. He sings, "Lah-lah!"
- The third can be a character from Sweden who only agrees. He says, "Yah-yah!"
- The fourth can be a character who loves football games. He says, "Rah-rah!"

Puppets can be used for this activity. A lot of fun will ensue when the child asks the characters various questions and the puppet answers with the same sound or word over and over again. When asked if they want eat ice cream, the first puppet will cry "Wah-wah," the second will sing "La-lah!" and so forth. Young children love this type of humor. Why would someone cry or sing when asked if he wants ice cream? Have clients practice saying all four of the puppets' sounds. Do so even before he can utter R correctly. This work will develop a curiosity about the way in which each sound appears similar but is different. It will stimulate the client's auditory discrimination skills as he listens carefully to recognize the sounds.

Discrimination of Correct and Incorrect

The ultimate goal of auditory discrimination work is to teach the client to differentiate or *discriminate* between correct and incorrect productions of the R sound. At this point, the treating therapist begins to produce sounds *incorrectly*. This work is always done with R in isolation and words, and sometimes with R in phrases, sentences and conversation. Such work teaches the client to recognize the correct R sound and its deviations. Auditory discrimination of correct and incorrect productions begins with gross distortions and progresses to fine ones. This final task, recognizing fine differences in productions of R, is the most difficult one. It is the auditory skill that is most critical for a successful outcome.

GROSS DIFFERENCES

Gross differences include obvious substitutions, complete omissions, and widely gross distortions of R. Early training can be done with repetitions of the same word multiple times. A therapist might repeat the word *rain* twenty times and say *wain* or *pain* as a substitution periodically. The client's job is to identify those few times when the therapist makes the mistake. In this way, the client hears far more correct productions than incorrect ones, and the wrong ones will stand out from the list. When he notices the error, she responds immediately to his correct identification. "You caught me! I said *wain* and you caught me. I should have said *rain*." This work helps train the ear to hear a correct R production, and it helps him to listen hard for deviations from it.

FINE DIFFERENCES

Once a client can make gross auditory discriminations of correct and incorrect sounds produced by the therapist, he is ready to move on to more refined listening work. Toward this end, we discontinue the use of substitution and omissions and concentrate on distortions. The distortions become more subtle and harder to recognize over time. We use the same types of activities as above. This process trains the ear to recognize increasingly finer distortions of the R sound, and it tunes the ear to greater precision. At this level of training, it is necessary for the speech and language pathologist to be able to make a perfect R sound, as well as many other R sounds with subtle and somewhat tricky distortions. The therapist should strive toward making the distortions similar to the client's distortion. The idea is to make this listening work increasingly difficult as the client is mastering his auditory discrimination skills. We are training his ear to hear these fine differences and to begin to hear how his own sound is wrong.

COMPARING FINE DIFFERENCES

Once a client has begun to hear the difference between a correct R and its subtle distortions, we can begin to compare and contrast them. The best way to do this is to ask the client to listen while you produce a correct R and then a distortion. Ask him to continue listening while you produce a string of eight or ten productions, weaving back and forth from good productions to bad ones. Slow down your utterances and stretch out the models. Make a continuous flow of sound as you slowly glide from one to another so the client can hear the changes that cause the distortions. Allow ample time. Remember, we are not testing him. We are training his ear to listen and identify correct and incorrect sound models. We help him hear gross distortions first, and over time, we may help him make increasingly finer discriminations.

Model-Response

The greatest auditory training tool we have in R therapy is our own production of the sound. Therapists provide models to which clients respond by imitation. We call this the *model-response*. A client's correct response to our model is a clear indication that his auditory discrimination skills are well-developed and he can hear the model well. But the opposite is *not* true. A client's incorrect response does not mean that his auditory discrimination skills are poor. It simply means that he cannot say the sound himself. A client can have perfect auditory discrimination of R and still be unable to pronounce it correctly.

When providing a correct model of R, therapists must learn to exaggerate the model without distorting it. The modeled sounds need to be big and over articulated. The therapist's mouth should be open as wide as possible for interoral viewing but not too wide that sound distortion results. The therapist should model production of the sound slowly and carefully, yet loudly and clearly. This production should make the sound of R stand out to the client like none he has ever heard before. It should be majestic. This grand model is where we start because it draws the client's auditory attention to the salient features of the correct acoustic quality of R. Do not let a client's R therapy fail simply because you are not modeling the sound with grandeur and distinction. The client is depending upon you to make this sound magnificently so that his ear will be well-trained. We model R correctly hundreds of times for our clients to imitate, so make sure you are performing them well. Again, if you cannot produce a correct R sound, refer the client to someone who can. And if you are working in an environment with a dialectal R sound that is somewhat different than your own, learn the standard for your area and use that as well. Then you will have to make a decision regarding which R to teach. Consult with other therapists in your area for advice and make a single decision for the approach you will make in your clinic or school district. Get parental input.

Amplification

A slight amount of amplification can help develop good auditory awareness and discrimination of R for any of the auditory activities in this chapter. Amplification can be achieved through use of a wide variety of equipment, from simple homemade devices to expensive amplification systems. The idea is to make listening tasks more interesting and easier to attend with sound that is a little louder. We are not talking about volumes that will damage a client's ears. Use amplification that works simply to make target sounds stand out.

THE HANDS

By far, the cheapest and most readily available amplification system is hands. To amplify her speech models, a therapist cups her own hands behind one or both of the client's ears as she pronounces sounds. The hands capture more sound than the ear alone, as if the client had extremely large external ears. The client's own hands also can be used behind his ears to hear the therapist's models. Or ask the client to cup one hand behind one of his ears, and the other hand in front of his mouth to hear an amplified version of his own sounds. When he utters a sound, it will reflect off the hand in front of his mouth and be captured by the hand behind his ear. The result will be slight yet significant amplification of his productions.

TUBES

Rubber, vinyl or cardboard tubes are an inexpensive way to amplify sound. Any tube can extend from the therapist's mouth to the client's ear, and flexible ones can extend from the client's own mouth to his own ear. Amplification through a tube will be strong. Hard plastic tubes amplify more than flexible plastic or cardboard ones. Use rubber tubing, vinyl tubing, plastic tubing, paper towel rolls, and so forth. Buy vinyl tubing inexpensively by the foot at hardware, plumbing or aquarium supply stores. Most can be cut into smaller pieces with a decent pair of scissors.

HOUSEHOLD OBJECTS

Bowls, cups and jars also make excellent low-tech amplification tools. Ask the client to make sound into the object as he tips the open end toward his face and ears. Little babies always do this once they discover how to blow bubbles and make other sounds into their cups or bowls at the end of a meal. Use little cereal bowls, large lightweight mixing bowls, stacking cups, large plastic jars, plastic or paper drinking cups or metal pots.

BOXES

Boxes of all shapes and sizes make good amplification devices for little or no cost. Use smaller boxes at the face, as described for household objects above, or have the client sit completely inside a large stove or refrigerator box to amplify sound all around him. Medium-size boxes can be placed directly over the head.

AMPLIFICATION DEVICES

A few items have been devised specifically to amplify sound. The TalkBack® device is an old-fashioned and inexpensive speech training tool that is still available today. Made of lightweight plastic, it looks like an elongated bowl that is curved into the shape of a big telephone receiver. It fastens loosely on one ear and extends to the mouth, like a wide hollow tube open along one side. Another is the HearPhone®. It looks like an earphone headset with long, clear plastic cups that are fastened to each earpiece and that extend down toward the mouth. Sound made by the client is captured by these long cups and directed to the ears. HearPhones were developed for singers to help them listen to the sound of their own voice as they rehearse.

TOYS

Some toys make excellent amplification tools. For example, many toy stethoscopes are constructed with tubes that lead from the ears to the round piece on the end. Use them by placing the earpieces in the client's ears and making sound into the other end. Sound can be made into the stethoscope by client or therapist.

HIGH-TECH EQUIPMENT

High-tech devices can be used to amplify sound. A basic tape recorder with an attached microphone and headset makes a decent amplification system if it is made of of good components. The client wears the earphones and listens to sound produced into the microphone by either the therapist or himself. We are not talking about recording the client and then listening to the recording. Instead, have the client use the earphones to listen to himself while he is speaking. The classic Auditory Trainer® is an outstanding high-tech tool for sound amplification. The trainer consists of a microphone, amplifier and set of earphones. The beauty of the auditory trainer is that it is constructed of pristine audio equipment. Sound can be adjusted by volume and frequency. Some classrooms and therapy rooms are fitted with amplification systems designed to amplify the teacher's speech to one child or the entire class. See if you can get training on how to use it if one is available at your school or clinic setting. Professional recording equipment, if available, also makes a great tool for auditory training because sound can be changed in a multitude of ways.

Auditory Bombardment
Auditory bombardment is a technique borrowed from phonological literature. It concerns the presentation of multiple examples of target sounds in words spoken by the therapist to a client who is engaged in a quiet activity. For example, a therapist might read a list of eight words that all end in similar R sounds—*bar, car, far, jar, star, tar, char* and *bizarre*. The words are spoken slowly and deliberately. Slight amplification is used to enhance the experience. The quiet activity is used to maximize the time a client can spend listening. Quiet activities that are appropriate for auditory bombardment include playing with Silly Putty®, clay or PlayDough®; coloring in a coloring book; constructing a puzzle; or placing stickers on a page. The idea is to give the client an opportunity to listen to the correct production of R multiple times as it occurs in a specific position of words while his hands are engaged in a quiet activity. The word list can be read one time through or several times in a row while the client is quietly engaged. Auditory bombardment can be used at all stages of R therapy. It's an excellent way to accustom the client to the correct production of R. The client is required to make no pronunciations throughout this activity. His job is simply to listen.

Imitation of the Client
A perfect model of R is not the only auditory stimulation necessary in successful therapy. Therapy models can be used to even greater advantage when we imitate our client's incorrect productions. This is called *echoing* or *mutual imitation*. By echoing or imitating a client's incorrect production, we mirror back to him an exact copy of his mispronunciation. We are modeling the error in order to help the client hear the problem, not to shame or belittle him. It is done to help him discover differences between correct R and his personal deviation.

In order for this technique to work, a client's sound error must be imitated by the therapist exactly as he makes it. Imitate the sound casually and without warning. For example, "You said . . ." Then pause. The client may be stunned as it dawns on him you are imitating his error. Pretend you do not know what the problem is. "What's wrong?" Allow time for the client to process the event, and then draw him into a discussion about it. Help the client learn to use you for feedback about how he is making his error sound.

Most clients find this work fascinating and accept it without question. Occasionally, a client will feel bad about this technique because he feels he is being mocked or kidded unfairly. When this occurs, clearly apologize for your insensitivity. Remember, rapport is an important element of successful R therapy. Tell the client that you did not mean to make fun of him. Explain that you wanted to help him hear the way he is saying the sound. Then drop it and backtrack to a secure place of trust. At some point later, ask, "May I repeat what you just said? I'd like you to hear it." Most clients develop a curiosity to hear this production once they get over their discomfort. They begin to understand what you are doing and why you are doing it. Discussion at this time helps many clients air their feelings about this error sound. I have seen many teary eyes during this activity, not because the client is hurt, but because he realizes that he has finally found someone who truly understands his problem. This is a huge relief to many clients. Work like this can bond the therapist and client like no other, when approached in the right way and at the right time. Modeling the client's error is one of the final solutions for helping him develop his auditory skills to maximum capacity for auditory training.

Vocal Synchrony
Another one of the most powerful techniques for stimulating good auditory discrimination of the R sound is based upon a process called *vocal synchrony*, when two or more people make the same sound at the same time. It's a process that appears during the earliest stage of infant vocal development, and it functions to develop primitive listening and imitation skills. For example, when a baby under four months of age coos, the attending adult might imitate the sound back to the child by saying it at the same time. We are all familiar with the coos and goos of adults as they talk to tiny babies. The adult matches the baby's sound by quality, pitch, resonance, loudness, length and vowel. In so doing, the adult creates a moment of time in which both he and the child are producing approximately the same sound. While the adult may be making the sound for fun or as a way to play with the child, this experience has a powerful impact on developing the infant's auditory system. The infant makes discoveries about the similarities between his vocalizations and those of another person. He begins to understand that he and another person can say the same thing at the same time. The experience stimulates him to attend to his own vocalizations and to compare them with sounds made by others.

A synchronous vocal experience can have the same effect on the client who is learning R. As the client produces and holds his distorted R sound, the therapist matches the sound precisely and simultaneously. This is like singing together, only we are making simultaneous phonemes. The acoustic mirror image of the client's sound begins to train his ear to hear his own sound in new ways as it is spoken by another person. Within a short period of time, the client will begin to hear his error. Now, we ask him to change oral shape in various ways. As he does, we change our sound with him so the two sounds continue to match. We demonstrate to the client exactly what he sounds like as he alters his oral position. This tunes his ear as he explores new oral positions. Synchronous production of R sounds is a powerful tool in auditory training. It takes the client's error outside of himself and puts it on display for him to observe visually and through auditory means.

Prolongation

Prolongation—lengthening out in time—of a target sound offers our clients the opportunity to focus the auditory system on the model. Typically, when a syllable or word containing R is spoken, the event happens in a split second. The sound comes and goes almost at once. Further, the swiftly spoken phoneme cannot be retrieved or held for observation. The prolongation of target sounds gives clients time to hear them for better awareness and discrimination. Prolongation of R by the therapist should be used heavily in the early stages of therapy when the client is first learning to make the sound. It also should be used intensively by the client and therapist together when the client is fine-tuning the sound later in the program. Prolongation of R to tune the ear should be a regular and consistent part of all R therapy programs.

Sound Bending

Sound bending is designed to help clients learn to reshape the oral mechanism for correct production of R while engaging in synchronous prolongations of R sounds. A client makes his incorrect R sound and holds it. The therapist matches the sound and produces it with synchronization. Then the therapist slowly begins to change, or bend, the sound by changing minute aspects of jaw, lip or tongue position. The client's work is to follow the therapist's lead and bend his sound in the same way. The therapist might give as instruction as follows, "I am going to make your sound. I want you to do it with me. While I am holding my sound, I am going to change it slightly by moving my tongue. Listen as my sound changes, and try to move your tongue and change the sound in the same way." Through this process, the client begins to learn how to alter his jaw, lip and tongue position to change the sound.

In the absence of oral-motor deficit, clients will be able to make these changes right away, although they may need time to play around with a wide variety of oral movements before they can figure out how to make the specific one you are demonstrating. Therefore, do not worry if the client begins to make widely erratic sounds. He needs this experimentation to figure out how oral movements alter sound productions. Imitate the client's oral movements to show him how the sounds can match. Continue to encourage him to do what you are doing. If oral-motor problems have been overlooked, this activity will reveal them. Sound bending is done regularly over the weeks of therapy. Ultimately, the sound bends away from the original incorrect sound and toward a correct R sound. Sound bending is enhanced with slight amplification.

Listening to the Hardest Words

Clients who are committed to learning to say R correctly often arrive with an agenda to learn certain words that cause them grief because they occur frequently. A client might be concerned that he cannot pronounce the words *world* or *earth* during geography or social studies classes. Another child may be having a hard time saying his own name or that of his best friend. A third student may be embarrassed because he cannot be understood when asked his age: *fourteen*. Another client may be very anxious about an upcoming oral bookreport on *James and the Giant Peach* by Roald Dahl because of the impossible pronunciation of the author's name.

Clients like these usually want to learn their problematic words months before they are ready. In fact, some clients arrive the first day of therapy and announce that they have come to learn these specific words. This matter is further complicated when parents think this is the purpose of therapy and want us to address these words from the start.

In these cases, I discuss what I call "The Hardest Words in the World." If we have begun a notebook of our work (see chapter 12), then I turn to the very last page of the notebook, insert a page at the end, and on the top write "The Hardest Words in the World." Then I begin to list the words he has mentioned. I inform the client that this is where we are going to list the words that are so hard that they will be the very last words he learns. I explain that when he has completely mastered everything in the book, including these most difficult words, he will be almost done with therapy. We talk about these words and their relevance in the client's life, and we add newly discovered words to the list throughout the course of therapy.

The words clients have the most difficulty with usually contain both R and L: *world, girl, squirrel, early, pearl, yearly,* and so forth. Also, most clients have particular vowels that cause them trouble with R, so list words with them as well. After the words are written, ask the client to say them the best way he can. Then tell him in clear terms that he cannot say them correctly. Don't tell him he said them pretty well or that he did a good job. Give him correct, simple and honest feedback. Say, for example, "Nope. That's not it. It's going to be a while until you can say that word correctly." Understand ahead of time that the client will fail miserably on these pronunciations. Empathize with him about how truly difficult they are. "That word is almost impossible to say!"

This idea is included in this chapter on auditory stimulation because the client's list of hardest words is an excellent set to use for listening exercises. Why? The client will be highly motivated to learn them and he will listen hard to your pronunciation of them. The list usually contains multisyllabic words. So make sure to speak them slowly and to draw them out one syllable at a time. Overexaggerate, over-pronounce and make R stand out. Return to these words time and again throughout treatment so the client can remember what he is aiming for. Reference these words each time he learns a new skill, to see if any of them contain R in the phonetic environment he has just learned. In addition to training his ear, the client's attempts at these words periodically throughout therapy will help him discover how well he is progressing.

Listening to Connected Speech
Perhaps the most difficult of the exercises is listening for R in connected speech. The therapist might read a paragraph or short story that contains R sounds. The client then is asked to respond to R sounds in a certain way. For example the client might snap his fingers or put a tally mark on a paper each time he hears an R. The activity might be made more difficult by producing some of the R sounds incorrectly. Now the client must recognize that an R sound was present and that it was made incorrectly. He can make one mark for correct R's and another one for incorrect R's. This work perhaps is best used later in therapy, when the client's ears are well-tuned. It is a nice break from production work at those later stages.

It is difficult because the client must listen to the content of the piece and its phonemes simultaneously.

Auditory Fatigue

Auditory fatigue is a fascinating phenomenon in articulation therapy. It's a weakening or breakdown in one's ability to make good auditory judgements that occurs after a length of time in a session or after a certain number of trials have taken place. Auditory fatigue appears more quickly when therapy is scheduled at the end of a long day or when the client is tired. It is seen more frequently in clients enrolled in individual therapy sessions, because the number of responses made per unit of time is much greater than that which occurs in group therapy. We see auditory fatigue in all types of articulation therapy, but it seems to be especially prevalent in R therapy. This is probably because of the refined nature of the acoustic properties of R.

When auditory fatigue occurs in R therapy, it is as if the part of the brain responsible for making acoustic judgements about the sound simply shuts down. The client may be moving along nicely and saying many R sounds well. Then *bam!* His skill shuts down. He can say the sound correctly no more. He can't hear it, nor can he arrange his mouth to say it. The system will come back to life after a period away from this work. Thus, therapists must arrange activities accordingly.

Arrange your work with little mental breaks. A simple two or three minute discussion on another topic can be sufficient to restore auditory discrimination ability. However, if after a significant break the client still cannot perform well, it is time to recognize that the production work should end for the day. Try to pace your activities so that auditory fatigue is avoided.

The other fascinating thing about auditory fatigue is that it also occurs in speech and language pathologists. A therapist's good judgement about correct and incorrect R productions often wanes during a late Friday afternoon appointment at the end of a long week. We hear so many different R sounds throughout a week that we can no longer tell which is correct. At these times, it is best to steer therapy in another direction. Use the time to engage in other rapport-building or logistical activities. This is a good time to talk about schedule changes for upcoming holidays. Or ask the client how he thinks he is doing. Sit back and listen. You probably will learn things that will help you in your next session. Also, use this time to listen to parents and their perception of progress. Afterward, think about altering your schedule so that your auditory fatigue does not interfere with the client's program.

Auditory stimulation will cause many clients to produce a new, correct R sound. This is great! It means that auditory input has proven to be the primary stimulation technique needed to change the client's pronunciation. There is no need to add any other type of stimulation to the program. Auditory stimulation has been the key to unlocking the door of good pronunciation. The initial R sound has been learned and the client is ready to move on to more advanced stages of production work. If auditory stimulation alone has not done the trick, it is time to add oral-motor work into the mix.

5 — *Summary* —

- Auditory stimulation trains the ear to hear productions of R. It is recognized as the most important avenue of stimulation for articulation training.

- Auditory stimulation alone can be sufficient to remediate an incorrect R in many clients. Thus, auditory stimulation usually is included early in treatment.

- Auditory stimulation can be done first, last or simultaneously with techniques to facilitate oral position.

- Some clients are unable to discriminate R until after they learn to produce it.

- Most therapy for R is initiated with exercises to help clients think about R as a phonetic unit in oral speech. Some clients learn this during a regular classroom reading and pre-reading activities.

- Auditory discrimination training teaches clients to recognize the presence or absence of R in words and to identify position of R in words.

- The most important work of auditory training is to teach clients to discriminate between correct and incorrect productions of R. This training begins with gross and ends with fine differences in R.

- Minimal-pair words teach recognition of sound differences in single words.

- Amplification makes R salient and draws the client's auditory attention to R.

- Synchronistic vocal production opens the ear to new sound.

- Prolongation of sound allows ample time to hear phoneme productions.

- Auditory bombardment familiarizes the ear to the correct sound of R.

- Sound bending teaches a client to change his distorted sound by following the therapist's lead as she alters oral position during slow production of the sound.

- Listening to prevalent hard words early in therapy motivates clients to stay involved for the long haul. We call these "The Hardest Words in the World."

- Listening to connected speech teaches a client to attend to the sound of R while his mind is also engaged in content.

- Auditory fatigue is a breakdown in the ability to make good auditory judgements. It occurs in clients and therapists after a certain length of treatment, which should be paced to avoid it. Non-auditory activities help to refresh the listening apparatus.

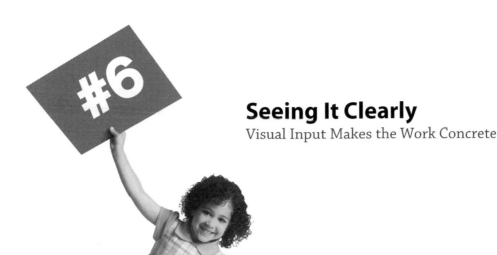

Seeing It Clearly
Visual Input Makes the Work Concrete

Visual input is the second most common form of stimulation during articulation therapy, although it is undervalued for its importance and often ignored in discussions about articulation therapy. Showing clients what to do with their mouths is a rock solid method of teaching a correct R with visual stimulation. Visual stimulation also includes the use of arm and hand gestures, facial expressions, mirrors, orthographic symbols and other graphic aids.

Visual input about oral position can help many clients learn to say R with almost no other teaching methods. These clients are able to translate what they see with their eyes into what to do with their mouths because they possess a highly organized sense of oral position and they have excellent integration between visual perception and oral-movement skills. Clients who can match oral position to a visual model usually are able to produce a correct R within a session or two. These are some of the dream clients who move quickly through treatment. The tools of visual stimulation are offered in this chapter. They can be the glue that holds together an entire R program.

Live Visual Models

The most common way to provide a visual model of R is for the therapist to model the sound—the *live visual model*. The client is asked to watch the therapist's mouth carefully as she makes an R sound. Since it is hard to see inside the mouth, the therapist usually opens the mouth wide and exaggerates the tongue movements without distorting the sound. For example, when modeling a Tip R, the therapist maintains the open position while sweeping the tongue tip up and back in a grand motion toward the velum. The movement is done slowly, and the action is repeated several times so the client can see. The therapist models the action and produces an acoustically correct R. Although either R can be modeled this way, the Tip R is far easier to see with a live model.

Live models require that a client is willing and able to look directly at the therapist's face and into her mouth. Most clients do this willingly, of course. A few clients are unwilling or unable to look in another person's mouth because of visual attention and tracking problems, general attention and organization problems, and the like. Some clients think it is "gross" to look closely into another person's mouth, especially an adult mouth. Some even feel like vomiting at the thought. The following ideas may help:

- Make sure your breath is fresh! Brush your teeth and your tongue before R clients if possible. Keep mints on hand.
- Give the client an excuse to look into an adult's mouth, like to count the teeth or see the fillings.
- Allow a client to glance quickly into the adult's mouth and then to look away and concentrate at a mirror image of his own mouth.
- Place a candy or mint on the tongue to make the process of looking into another person's mouth more acceptable.
- Shine a flashlight into the mouth to make viewing more interesting.
- Use tongue depressors to make the experience more clinical.
- Peer into the mouth while chewing dry snack foods (crackers, cookies). Also, stick out the tongue while it is coated with mashed food. Talk about the inappropriateness of this behavior outside of the therapy room. Then use it to discover aspects of tongue movement. These actions are considered "gross" and therefore quite appealing to most young clients.

Once the live model is given and the sound of R is produced, the client is asked to imitate it with his own mouth. If a client can learn the oral movements necessary for R with the live model, there is no need to offer further models or more invasive stimulation techniques. Treatment can progress to more advanced levels of the program.

Visual Discrimination

The way R looks must be visually discriminated from the way the other glides look. Therefore, all four glides—W, L, Y and R—must be practiced and viewed together in one activity. In the previous chapter, we discussed the development of four characters with the names *Wah, Lah, Yah* and *Rah,* and we assigned sounds for them to say. This is a great idea to help young children pay attention to the subtle movement variations of these four sounds. The similarity of their names, sounds and words encourages the children to peer into the therapist's mouth in order to see how they are different. Older clients can do the same type of work without the characters, simply by writing each nonsense word on paper and asking the client to circle the one he sees you say. Add mirrors to the activity to help the children learn to visually discriminate the way they make the four sounds. Visual discrimination of the similarities and differences between the four glides is an important part of early therapy for most R clients. Many clients will discover their error on R while looking in the mirror this way, and some will figure out how to say it correctly with this simple method.

Hand Models

A second ready form of visual input is to use hand models. The hand can model either the Tip R or the Back R. Practice these several times here before using them with clients.

TIP R
To model the Tip R, the hand is positioned with fingers extended and the palm up. The fingertips represent the tongue tip, and the heal of the hand represents the tongue back. The client is asked to watch carefully as the therapist slowly says a Tip R while modeling the tongue's movements with her hand. The fingertips are lifted and curled back to replicate the upward and rearward curling of the tongue tip. The therapist can model a vocalic or a consonantal Tip R, as long as the hand movements correspond exactly with the movements of the tongue.

BACK R
To model the Back R, the hand is positioned with fingers extended and the palm down. The fingertips represent the tongue tip, and the wrist represents the tongue back. The client is asked to watch carefully as the therapist slowly says a Back R, modeling the tongue's movement with her hand. The wrist elevates to replicate the upward elevation of the tongue back. The therapist can model a vocalic or a consonantal Back R, as long as the hand movements correspond exactly with the movement of the tongue. Please note that the hand model of Back R is a *gross* representation of its tongue movement. As the reader will recall, the Back R actually is made with the lateral backs high and stationary and the middle back tensing up and forward. If the client needs a refined definition of back elevation to produce a correct R, the hand model will not suffice. Specific tactile and proprioceptive stimulation techniques will have to be used, and a different visual model will be needed. These are discussed later.

A hand model can be the key to understanding tongue movements for R. If so, no additional stimulation techniques will be necessary, and R can be practiced immediately.

Oral Movement with Hand and Arm Gestures

Arm and hand gestures and facial expressions can facilitate a client's understanding of the R phoneme. Like an orchestra conductor, the speech and language pathologists can use her arm and hand gestures to mark rhythm and timing of productions, as well as syllable, stress, intonation, loudness and prolongation of sound or syllable. For example, long sweeping gestures can help clients stretch out their hurried utterances so that they have time to reach the tongue into position. Facial expressions are used to reinforce good productions and to halt the client in the middle of bad ones. There are no set procedures for the use of these visual indicators. Each therapist must look to her own skills, and design ones that are appropriate to personality and circumstance.

Puppets

Puppets can be used, to a limited extent, in modeling tongue position for R. A puppet with an attached tongue must be selected, and the tongue must be able to house the therapist's finger or hand. Usually these puppets have big mouths that open wide. If the tongue can house a finger and its mouth opens wide enough, the Back R can be modeled. The Back R is used because the finger can hump up and back to make the tongue do the same. A Tip R is more difficult. The finger has to be in the puppet upside-down to make the tip elevate and retract. Most puppets are not this accommodating. Some puppets are large enough that the therapist's whole hand enters the tongue. With such a puppet, either the Tip R or the Back R can be modeled.

The right puppet can be really fun in therapy, especially with small children. A puppet can model oral positions, and it can be used as a character to talk about how to make an R. A puppet can make all kinds of funny mistakes that get the kids involved in the process. An inexpensive yet highly effective puppet model can be made with a sock. Put your hand inside a sock and pretend that it is a big tongue. A free-floating tongue can be hugely entertaining for children and can help demonstrate the tongue movements necessary for R production. Make sure the sock fits snugly so that the hand movements underneath are obvious. A big, floppy sock will not do.

Schematic Illustrations

Schematic illustrations (line drawings) can be used as visual input regarding tongue position for R production and for training specific oral-motor techniques. A pictographic image is an excellent way to explain these things. In fact, an illustration can be more effective than a photograph because it can be drawn specific to the features being taught. Draw with bold lines, and label parts to be highlighted. Three samples are offered below.

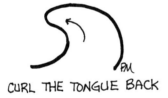

Fig. 6.1. Illustration to teach a client how to curl the tongue to make a Tip R.

Fig. 6.2. Illustration to teach a client how to brush the tongue along the middle.

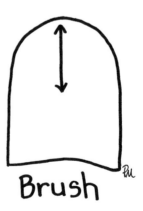

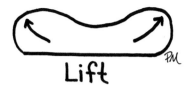

Fig. 6.3. Illustration to teach a client how to lift the sides of the tongue.

Additional schematic illustrations of the tongue movements necessary to make a Tip R and a Back R are included in the chapters that describe these oral-motor activities.

Mirrors

Mirrors are used to give visual feedback to clients about their own jaw, lip and tongue movements. A visual reflection almost always helps clients figure out better ways to move the mouth, especially the tongue. The following ideas are offered to help in mirror work:

- Ask clients to open their mouths wide.
- Use lip retractors to draw a client's lips out of the way for better oral viewing and to make the work more interesting. (See chapter 7.)
- Shine flashlights into the mouth for a better view and to make the work more interesting.
- Keep mirrors of various sizes at hand. Big mirrors can be fun, but small handheld mirrors are best for mouth viewing.
- Discontinue mirror work if it causes too much distraction. Some clients use a mirror to look at everything else in the room except their own mouth. Bring a mirror out periodically to see if these clients are ready to handle one, and use it when they are.
- Give adolescents the necessary silent moment to investigate their hair, skin or makeup in the mirror. Then simply pull them back on task with a direction.

Auditory Feedback from Visual Model

Clients should be asked to produce sound as they are moving their mouths around in response to visual models or mirrored visual feedback. The acoustic quality of the sound they produce at these times helps you hear if they are benefitting from visual input. If the client is beginning to make better sound, you know that the visual input you are providing is being helpful.

Vocabulary of Visual Input

The vocabulary we use to describe our visual models is extremely important. Our words direct a client's visual attention to the features we are trying to alter. It may seem silly to spell out the vocabulary for visual models. However, countless hours of therapy can be wasted when clients do not know what their therapists are talking about. A client's inability to position the mouth correctly for R may be due to poor oral control, but it could be a problem of unshared vocabulary.

When vocabulary words or phrases are not mutually understood, it is difficult for clients to comply with verbal directions. A client cannot "lift up the sides of the tongue" if he does not know where they are. Therapy for R is full of such directions. Thus, clients must have a vocabulary to support these visual images. Specific labels straighten out this confusion and help assure success.

Teaching the vocabulary of visual input does not need to take up a lot of therapy time. It only takes a moment to teach the meaning of a vocabulary word or phrase. "Lift up the sides of your tongue. Do you know where the sides are? Let me draw you a picture.... Do you see this part and that part? Those are the sides." These little asides help the client understand the vocabulary of visual image, which enables faster and better success in R therapy.

THE PARTS OF THE MOUTH

- Face
- Mouth
- Lips
- Top Lip
- Bottom Lip
- Sides (Corners) of the Lips
- Cheeks
- Teeth
- Front Teeth
- Back Teeth
- Top Teeth

- Bottom Teeth
- Jaw
- Tongue
- Tip of the Tongue
- Back of the Tongue
- Blade of the Tongue
- Sides of the Tongue
- Middle of the Tongue
- Roof of the Mouth
- Velum
- Throat

DIRECTION WORDS FOR ORAL MOVEMENT

- Up
- Down
- High
- Low
- Left
- Right

- Inside the Mouth
- Outside the Mouth
- Front of the Mouth
- Back of the Mouth
- Side of the Mouth

ACTION WORDS OF ORAL MOVEMENT

- Pull
- Push
- Lift
- Lower
- Stretch

- Curl
- Hump
- Spread
- Tighten
- Relax

Creative Visual Imagery
Most therapists develop a vocabulary for the mouth that is more picturesque than what is described above. For example, a place where the tongue humps can be called a "hill." Its depressed area can be called a "valley." Sometimes clients are asked to make a "bowl" or a "cup" with the tongue. Imaginative visual images help clients understand the tongue's position for production of R.

Visual imagery can be mundane or wild. A classic example of creative visual imagery is to name the lingual appendage "Mr. Tongue." Therapists create stories about him to help clients understand oral movement. For example, Mr. Tongue lives in a "house" (the mouth) that has a "roof" (the palate), "walls" (the cheeks), and a "door" (the teeth). The door can open and close (the mouth opens and closes). Mr. Tongue exercises in his house (moves around), dances (moves back and forth), works out with his punching bag (taps the velum), and paints or washes his walls and roof (rubs the tongue tip against the cheeks and palate).

Visual imagery like this is designed to capture the imaginations of our clients, and to help them grasp concepts that otherwise may be too abstract. Visual imagery can get too sappy and useless, of course, but it can be a wonderful stimulant to an otherwise dull routine when used sparingly.

Orthographic Symbols
Visual stimulation in R therapy also includes the use of orthographic symbols to draw the client's attention to the concept of R. These can be powerful. Orthographic symbols are the written alphabet letters, including A/a, B/b, C/c, and so forth. The written upper and lowercase orthographic symbols R/r are used throughout the entire process of therapy as a visual reference for the sound being learned. The written letter is a concrete symbol upon which the client can place his attention. It becomes a focal point for each day's work. This is an important element of therapy, especially for young children. The permanent nature of the visual symbol is critical. Think about this: When we say a sound, it is here one moment and gone the next. Oral speech disappears into the auditory environment never to be retrieved again. But the written symbol becomes a permanent part of the visual environment. By writing the symbol down, we make the sound concrete and, therefore, easier to conceptualize and remember. This is especially necessary with our clients who have poor auditory skills.

The easiest and most effective way to center a client's visual attention on the concept of R is to draw it in the middle of a blank sheet of paper with a colorful marker. I like to begin my first session with "Why are you coming to see me?" When the client answers something about learning to say R, I then draw an R about two inches in height as they watch. Usually I put a circle around it, to help them see it as a complete concept. Sometimes I have the client draw it himself, and I ask him to draw a circle around it. But most children love to watch adults draw letters. By drawing it myself, I can attract the client's attention toward me and the topic. I begin with a plain R. Over time, I draw these letters with unusual fonts to capture their visual attention throughout therapy.

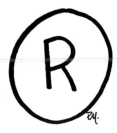

Fig. 6.5. R is written down to draw the client's attention.

The written symbol of every practiced word is written down in like manner. I like to write each word myself, even with older clients, so that I can pronounce and spell simultaneously. Over the years, I have developed a special skill: I write the words from right to left and upside-down so that the written work always unfolds correctly for the client across the table. Writing upside-down causes quite a buzz with my clients and their parents. It further focuses their visual attention on the process.

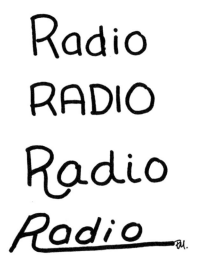

Fig. 6.6. Written words in large letters with interesting fonts and colorful markers draw the client's attention to the page and the concept of R.

Graphics Amplify Speech Features

Simple graphics can be used with orthographic symbols to remind a client of specific practice features. An arrow can be drawn to indicate that a sound should be prolonged. There is no limit to the creative ways in which therapists can design visual symbols and graphic elements to teach treatment concepts. Three samples are offered here:

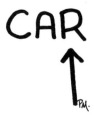

Fig. 6.7. To remind a client to say his good R sound at the end of certain words, write the words in large block letters and draw an arrow pointing toward the final R of each word.

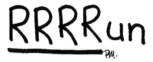

Fig. 6.8. Several R's can be written at the beginning of a word to highlight the sound. Draw a line under the sounds to indicate that the client should hold the sound.

Fig. 6.9. Draw a face with an open mouth in front of an R word when a client needs to remember to open his mouth wide before trying R.

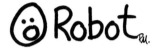

The Hope of Auditory and Visual Input
Auditory and visual stimuli are included early in R therapy in the hope that our clients will learn to pronounce a correct R sound without needing further input. Why? Because the auditory and visual work described so far is simple, safe and non-invasive. Easy clients will learn correct R with these methods alone. But the client with a longterm persistent R distortion usually needs much more than simple auditory and visual input to be successful. He needs specific tactile and proprioceptive stimulation. It is to these topics that we advance in our next two chapters.

Summary

- Visual input is an overlooked yet important part of successful R therapy.

- Some clients learn to say R with visual input only. They are able to translate what they see with their eyes into what to do with their mouths. These are dream clients who progress through therapy rapidly.

- Visual models are used to help clients see how the tongue moves into and out of position for R. The live, exaggerated model is the most common visual model.

- Hand gestures can be used to model the Tip R or the Back R. The hand model is a gross yet frequently effective representation of tongue movement.

- Puppets can be used to a limited extent to model tongue position for R. A puppet with an attached tongue must be selected, and the tongue must be able to house the therapist's finger or hand. A sock puppet on the hand to make a big tongue is a fun alternative to traditional puppets. Puppets are most useful in therapy when they become hapless participants also trying to learn R.

- Schematic illustrations provide specific visual information about the mouth, its parts and its movements.

- A mirror gives visual feedback about a client's own oral movements.

- Sound produced while imitating visual models allows us to hear the effectiveness of our visual input.

- The vocabulary of visual input must be shared between therapist and client for visual input to be effective. Take a moment periodically to teach key words.

- Creative visual imagery enlists a client's imagination in the treatment process. It can be wild and imaginative or scientific.

- Orthographic symbols are powerful. They help focus a client's attention on the topic phoneme. Orthographic symbols make the abstract concept of R concrete.

- Simple graphics are used along with orthographic symbols to remind clients of specific practice features.

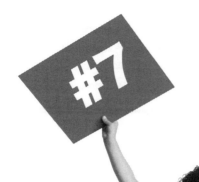

Positioning the Tongue for a Tip R
Methods to Achieve the Easy Grand Sweep

Are you ready to take your oral-motor therapy to new heights? The heart of successful R therapy lies in a client's ability to position the jaw, lips and tongue in ways that allow the correct acoustic quality of R to emerge. In this and the next chapter we shall describe the two methods of R production, Tip R and Back R, separately because the movements and the methods to achieve them are unique. We begin with the Tip R. It is simpler to describe, easier to see, more convenient to model, and less complicated to understand. It also is the R that most clients can learn with the least amount of difficulty.

We shall discuss the *cornerstone sound*, a client's first Tip or Back R that he produces correctly and that he can repeat consistently. The cornerstone R is the first one to which we can shout, "That's it!" The cornerstone sound is not necessarily the sound of R in isolation. In fact, few clients with longterm, persistent R distortion are able to learn an R in isolation first. It is too difficult. Instead, most of these clients learn either a Consonantal or Vocalic R, which means that their first R is part of a syllable. The cornerstone R is a Consonantal or a Vocalic R that contains a clear R tone at the apex of movement. It is not distorted by nasality, vocal quality, oral position or by adding other sounds to it. No matter if the client makes a Consonantal or a Vocalic R sound, there should be no doubt in your mind about the cornerstone R's perfect auditory quality at the apex. Pay very close attention to this first correct sound. It is the R upon which the rest of the client's program will be constructed.

Jaw, lip *and* tongue position are critical for successful production of both the Tip R and the Back R. But the biggest, far-reaching influence toward achieving the cornerstone sound comes from tongue position.

Do Not Say R
A few introductory comments must be written about the process of learning either a Tip or a Back R before we describe the techniques to acquire them. It is important that clients concentrate on oral movement through this process and that they just don't try to "say R." In fact, throughout the lessons of this and the next chapter, clients are explicitly told: "Do not say R." This is especially important for difficult clients. It is necessary to avoid attempts to say R, because to do so will cause most clients to resort to old, incorrect habits. In fact,

a client's continual attempts to say R usually retards his progress. Old movement patterns are so ingrained that they must be avoided for success. The client must learn to inhibit the familiar movement patterns while the new movement pattern is being facilitated.

Along this line, it is my habit to tell clients to forget everything they have ever learned about producing R before they begin. Clients are told that therapy will begin from scratch, as if they have never tried R before in their lives. They are told that the purpose of this fresh approach is to get their tongue to work better before they practice R again. "Forget about everything you have learned about R before. In fact, forget about R for now. Focus on what I am saying, and follow my directions. The more carefully you pay attention to what I am saying, and the more carefully you follow my directions, the easier this work will be and the faster you will get through it." Treatment progresses with the client thinking that he is doing mouth or tongue exercises. Phoneme R will be the final result, but the client will not be trying to make this happen. This is done to help him break old oral-movement habits and acquire new ones.

Learning the Tip R

The essential tongue movement needed for production of the Tip R is a sweeping up and back of the tongue tip so that it approaches but does not touch the velum. We have named it the *grand sweep*. Simultaneous to the upward and backward sweep is the relative depression of the middle sections of the tongue. As such, the tip leads the movement as it curls back. This gives the tongue its thinness and required level of tension. With elevation and curling of the tip comes elevation and curling of the sides, or lateral margins of the tongue, to form the rear-facing cave described in chapter 1.

Probably the greatest mistake therapists make in regard to the Tip R is to ignore it as a treatment option because of an antiquated view that it is not a proper R. The Tip R is normal and should be facilitated in treatment, especially when R has proven difficult to achieve. Facilitation of tongue position for the Tip R is achieved through visual, tactile and proprioceptive means.

Remember, we use the client's production of sound to judge his oral position. Use it liberally throughout the following. Also remember, that either a Consonantal or Vocalic R can be stimulated. These, as well as the isolated R and sequences with R are described here. In the following sections, we shall describe six methods for eliciting the Tip R:

1. The live visual model
2. The hand model
3. Tap into position
4. Slide into position
5. The external tactile cue
6. Guiding into position with resistance

The Live Visual Model

The visual model is the most common way to initiate Tip R therapy. It is the least invasive to the client, the easiest to model, requires the least amount of materials, and many clients can learn a Tip R simply from visual models alone. A live visual model is a way for a therapist to demonstrate correct oral position with her own mouth. Readers are encouraged to try each of these steps so that their meaning comes alive. These procedures are the essential ones for facilitating a Tip R.

1. Open your mouth wide (as wide as it will go), hold it open, and sweep the tip of your tongue up and back so that it heads toward but does not touch the velum. Do so in silence so that the client can focus on the movement and not the sound. A simple direction like, "Watch my tongue" will be enough to get the client's attention focused on your tongue.
2. Make a few comments about the tongue movement to make sure that the client's attention is drawn to the correct features. "Did you see what my tongue did? Right. It went up and back. Watch again."
3. Model the grand sweeping movement a few more times.
4. Then ask the client to imitate your oral movement. Say, "Can you do that? Can you make your tongue go up and way back?" As described above, do not ask him to say R at this point. You do not want him to try the sound, because he probably will make it his old way. You are teaching him the movement at this point, not the sound. Have him imitate the movement in silence.
5. Once the movement looks like it might be correct, ask him to make a sound while performing it. We can do this in four ways. Try all four to see that way will work for your client.

   - *Vocalic Tip R:* Some clients will learn to produce a Tip R in the vocalic position. Remember, the Vocalic R is made at the end of a syllable, after a vowel. Therefore, voice is made at the same time the tongue sweeps up and back.

     Have the client begin voicing while his mouth is open, and ask him to hold the sound as the tongue tip sweeps up and back. Again, do not ask him to say R. Simply encourage him to make a sound when his mouth is open, and to continue to make the sound while the tongue sweeps up and back. He will produce "Ah" with the mouth open, and he may produce R when the tongue hits its highest point. The vocalic production of /ɑɚ/ or Ah-R will result if he has done it right. This seems to be one of the simplest ways to learn the Tip R for both easy and difficult clients.
   - *Consonantal Tip R:* Some clients will learn to produce a Tip R in the consonantal position. Remember, the Consonantal R occurs before a vowel and opens a syllable. Therefore, voice is made *after* the tongue has swept up and back.

     Have the client open his mouth wide in silence. Ask him to elevate and curl his tongue tip in silence. Then ask him to begin voicing after the tongue has reached its highest point. Have him continue to voice as the tongue sweeps back down to the neutral position. Again, do not ask him to say R. Encourage him to make a sound when his tongue tip is high, and to continue to make the sound while the tongue tip sweeps down. He will say R when the tongue tip is high and "Ah" once it lowers. The consonantal production of /ra/ or R-Ah will result if he has done it right. This too seems to be one of the easiest ways to learn the Tip R for difficult clients.

- *Isolated Tip R:* Some clients will learn to produce a Tip R in the isolated position. Remember, the isolated R occurs when voice is produced only while the tongue tip is held in its highest position. I like to think of this as the pure acoustic sound of R. It represents the essence of the R sound in both the vocalic and consonantal production.

    Have the client open his mouth and curl his tongue tip up and back in silence. Then ask him to begin voicing once the tongue has reached its highest point. Have him maintain voice while he holds the tongue high in this position. Again, do not ask him to say R. Encourage him to make voice after his tongue tip attains its highest position. The client should stop voicing before lowering the tongue again. The sound of isolated R will result if the tongue position is correct and the tone is adequate. This is one of the hardest ways to learn the Tip R because the tongue's movements take place in silence.

- *Gross Vowel Sequences with Tip R:* Many clients will have to learn a Tip R in the same way that a baby does: moving the tongue up and down while voicing. Babies do this while cooing, but our clients do it simply while prolonging an open vowel.

    Ask the client to say "Ah" and to prolong it. While holding the vowel, ask him to sweep the tongue tip up and down toward and away from the velum in a repetitious sequence. Often, a good R will be heard intermittently as the tongue reaches its highest point. The production of /ararara/ will result if the client can make an appropriate movement of the tip toward the velum. This is a sloppy way to learn R but can be effective. The gross sweeping-back-and-forward action of the tongue tip causes the client to break away from his old tongue movement patterns and his attempts to say R. This action loosens the stiff tongue, and helps to tone up the floppy one. It also pulls the lips out of the way for those clients who habitually produce a W-for-R substitution. This is a great warm-up exercise, and it makes for a good homework assignment. Please note that many clients need to practice this gross sequence with Ah and R for a month or so prior to learning a consonantal, vocalic or an isolated R sound.

6. By this point you may have noticed that your client cannot prolong voice long enough to keep a steady stream of sound going while he performs the tongue movements of step 5. You also may notice that the voice sounds weak, muffled, nasalized or poorly projected. If so, back up and work for a while on prolonged vowels. Teach him to sit up straight, speak louder and to send his voice out so that it is strong and sits "in front" of the client. Work on vowels intermittently until the voice is strong enough to be maintained throughout the exercises in step 5. You may need to work on the strength of the voice for several weeks or months. A few clients will need to work on voice throughout their entire program.

7. The sound of R in the consonantal, vocalic, isolated or gross sequence should be pretty good at this point if the following conditions are being met:

   - The client is moving his tongue accurately
   - The client has attained an appropriate amount of tension in the tongue
   - Jaw and lip position have fallen into place without direct instruction
   - Voice and resonance are good

If a good R sound results from these methods, then you have taught a Tip R that should be celebrated and rehearsed. This is your client's cornerstone R sound! If a good R sound does not result from this basic method, move along to others.

The Hand Model

The hand model is an excellent way to expand your visual input. Use your own bare hand, a puppet with a tongue that can house a hand, or a sock placed on the hand to make a big tongue puppet. The following steps are recommended:

1. Hold out your hand, palm up and fingertips facing the client.
2. Explain that you are going to use your hand as a model of the tongue. "Let's pretend that my hand is a tongue. Here is the tip of the tongue [point to fingertips], and here is the back of my tongue" [point to heal of hand].
3. Explain that you are going to move your hand the same way that you move your tongue while saying R. Utilize one or more of the following four procedures.

   - *Vocalic R:* Hold the hand flat and say "Ah." Then slowly curl the fingertips up and back so they settle in position two inches above the heal of the hand. Curl your tongue up and back simultaneously. Produce voice throughout so Ah gradually changes into R. You will be saying /aɚ/, the Vocalic R sound.
   - *Consonantal R:* Curl the fingertips up and back so they settle in position two inches above the heal of the hand. Curl the tongue tip up and back to mirror the hand and say R. Then lower the fingertips and say "Ah." Do the exact same motion with your tongue so that R gradually changes into Ah. You will be saying /rɑ/, the Consonantal R sound.
   - *Isolated R:* Curl the fingertips up and back so they settle in position two inches above the heal of the hand. Maintain the position while you say the Tip R. This is the isolated R sound.
   - *Gross R Sequence:* Curl the fingertips up and down to mirror the tongue's movements as you say /ɑrɑrɑrɑ/. Make sure that the up-and-down movements of your fingers correspond with the up-and-down movements of your tongue.

4. Get verbal feedback from the client. Ask him if he watched what you did, and ask him to explain what he saw. Ask him what he heard and if he understood you were doing the same movement with both your hand and your tongue.

5. Ask the client to watch and listen again several times as you model with the hand and with the mouth.
6. Ask the client to imitate the hand motions with one of his own hands. Repeat several times until he does it well.
7. Ask him to do the same thing with his tongue that he did with his hand. Then ask him to do it with voice. If he can prolong voice throughout, he should say Ah and R in one or more of the sequences described in step 3.
8. If the client cannot prolong voice long enough to keep a steady stream of sound going while he performs the tongue movements, back up and work on sound prolongation for a while as described above. Then return to the hand and tongue practice as described above.
9. The sound of R should be pretty good at this point if the following conditions are met:

    - The client is moving his tongue accurately
    - The tongue has achieved an appropriate amount of tension
    - Jaw and lip position have fallen into place without direct instruction
    - Voice and resonance are good

If a good R sound results from a hand model, you have taught a Tip R that should be celebrated and rehearsed. This is your client's cornerstone R sound! If a good R sound does not result from this method, move along to others, or switch to a Back R.

Tap into Position

An excellent traditional technique to facilitate the consonantal form of the Tip R is a tapping exercise. We begin with the oral movements for L and end with an acoustically correct R. The following steps are required. It is strongly recommended that the reader try each step to understand them fully. Model each step clearly for the client to imitate. And consider using a simple schematic illustration throughout this activity in order to illustrate the points where the tongue tip should tap along the palate.

1. Ask the client to open his mouth wide and say "Lah" by lifting and lowering the tongue tip to the alveolar ridge. Have him say it loud and clear. Make sure the mouth is open wide and the up-and-down tongue movements of the tongue tip are clean and deliberate. The client should make the L sound with the tongue tip articulating with the alveolar ridge. If so, move to the next step. If L or the vowel is unclear or poorly articulated, backtrack and work on them until their articulation is excellent. Then move on to the next step.
2. Have client say "Lah" again with the mouth wide open. This time tap the tongue tip slightly back from, or posterior to, the alveolar ridge. The sound of L should still be recognizable but slightly distorted because the tongue-tip position on the palate is slightly posterior to where it should be for a good L.

3. Have the client say "Lah" again, but this time tap the tip even further back from the alveolar ridge—in the middle of the palate. The sound of L should be so distorted that it is nearly unrecognizable as an L. The sound is not L any longer. Neither is it R. It is a non-English palatal glide.
4. Have the client perform this movement again. Now, tap the tip of the tongue on the palate at the palatal notch, where the bony structure of the hard palate ends. This syllable may sound like "Rah." If not, have him smile broadly while performing this action. Do not tell him to say R. If the R sounds good, accept it and begin rehearsal. If not, move on to the next step.
5. Have the client stretch the tip even further back and tap it on the velum and repeat the action. The production may be a good Rah syllable. However, do not tell him to say R.
6. If any of these basic movement positions sounds good but not perfect, the slight distortion may be the result of positioning the tip too high. Ask the client to repeat his action and to curl up to the same place, but tell him not to touch the palate. See if he can curl up as if he were going to touch the palate but then stop short of doing so.

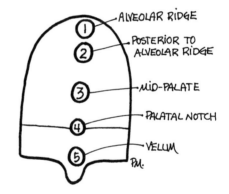

Fig. 7.1. Tap the tongue tip to each position to determine which will facilitate an acoustically correct R.

If a good R sound results from these methods, you have taught a Tip R that should be celebrated and rehearsed. This is your client's cornerstone R sound! If a good R sound does not result from this method consider having him repeat it with firmer contact of the tip to the various places along the midline of the palate. Also consider changing this exercise to be a vocalic or intervocalic production. A poor R will result if the client thickens and elevates the middle of the tongue while curling the tip up into the rear position. This is a common occurrence and requires that the client learn to curl without midline thickening, which is described later in this chapter.

Slide into Position
The *L-to-R slide* also uses L to stimulate the Tip R. It is an excellent traditional articulation method to teach R production. The following steps are suggested. Model each one clearly for the client to imitate. Draw a schematic to indicate the points of articulation along the midline of the palate.

1. Ask the client to elevate the tip of his tongue to the alveolar ridge and say "L." Ask him to hold the tip high and prolong this sound while his mouth is open wide.
2. Ask the client to prolong the sound while he slides his tongue tip back along the palate at midline, from the alveolar ridge to the velum. If tongue position and tension are good throughout, the sound of R should result somewhere along this midpalatal line. Usually, the sound becomes good as the tip approaches the palatal notch and deteriorates as it moves further back. Listen hard to find the right point, and experiment with more anterior and posterior positions until you find the right spot. A good R heard somewhere along this line should be recognized as such. It should be rewarded and rehearsed as the cornerstone sound. This will be a true isolated R sound. A poor R will result if the client thickens and elevates the middle of the tongue while curling the tip. This is a common occurrence and requires that the client learn to curl without midline thickening, which is described later.

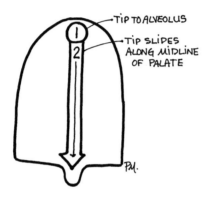

Fig. 7.2. Place tip on alveolus and slide back along midline of the palate while prolonging L.

3. Consider using the *Z-to-R slide* as an alternative slide method. Ask the client to say and prolong a Z sound and to hold the sound as he slides his tongue tip back toward the velum and along the midline of the palate. This method is a little more difficult to do than the L-to-R slide because it is harder to hold the voiced frication as the tip slides back along the palate. It is a great technique for some clients, however. If tongue position and tension are good throughout, the sound of R should result as the tongue tip reaches back somewhere along the midline of the palate. Usually, the sound becomes good as the tip approaches the palatal notch and deteriorates as it moves further back. Listen hard to find the right point, and experiment with more anterior and posterior positions until you find the right spot. This will be a true isolated R sound. Remember, do *not* ask the client to say R.

If a good R sound results from these methods, you have taught a Tip R that should be celebrated and rehearsed. This is your client's cornerstone R sound. If a good Tip R sound is not achievable with either the L-to-R or the Z-to-R slide, consider another method or switch to the Back R.

The External Tactile Cue

One of the most interesting techniques for assisting clients in positioning the Tip R is the *external tactile cue*. Exactly what the name suggests, it is the use of touch on the outside of the head to instruct or remind a client about a movement. In this case, tongue movement. The idea is to give the client information about where to position the tongue tip. Since the Tip R is made by elevating and curling back the tip, it ends up facing the back of the head. As such, a touch cue is given to the back of the head at the point where the therapist thinks the tip should face. The following steps are recommended:

1. Teach the client to elevate and curl the tongue tip toward the velum as described above.
2. Use one finger or thumb to press against the back of the head at the base of the occipital bone. This is the place on the outside of the head, just about directly behind the rear-facing tip. Tell the client to push his tongue tip toward that point by saying, "Push toward my finger."
3. Ask the client to produce sound while in this position. Do not ask him to say R. If tongue position is good, and enough tension is generated, a good R sound should result. If so, reward and rehearse this cornerstone sound.
4. If a good R sound does not result, change the position of your finger or thumb on the head. Some clients will produce a better sound if they angle the tip higher and some lower. If the sound is still poor, lift higher and repeat. Try lower positions the same way. Sometimes the oddest position will stimulate a correct R sound. For example, some clients achieve a correct R sound when the top of the head is pressed, or when a place above each ear is pressed. Experiment with these positions using the client's production to determine effectiveness of position.

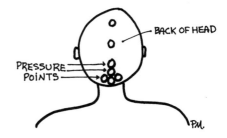

Fig. 7.3. Press on the outside of the back of the head in order to point the tongue tip toward the rear.

This technique has another benefit in addition to setting tip position. Some clients are able to turn the tip toward the back for a Tip R, but then are unable to generate enough tension throughout the tongue to achieve the correct acoustic quality for a good R. This external cue can help generate the required tension if the client is asked to "push" the tip toward the external point of stimulation.

Guiding and Thinning the Tongue

One of my favorite techniques uses a *dental floss holder* to guide the tongue into position for a Tip R. This is a tool for flossing the teeth. Its design makes an excellent tool for guiding the tongue into position for the Tip R. It uses the holder to provide resistance to the tongue tip as it curls up and back. The following steps are recommended.

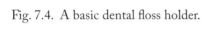
Fig. 7.4. A basic dental floss holder.

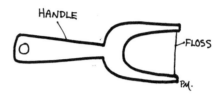

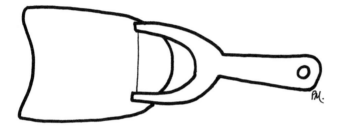

Fig. 7.5. Placement of the dental floss holder.

1. With the mouth open wide and the tongue out, place the dental floss holder on the tongue with the floss stretched across the blade. Provide the client with a paper towel for escaping saliva.
2. Ask the client to curl the tip up and "grab" the floss. Then ask him to pull the floss holder back into the mouth as far as he can. Tug slightly on the floss holder so that it provides a little bit of resistance to the client's rearward movement. This increases the tongue's muscular effort at the tip and increases thinning in the middle section. The tongue tip should curl up and carry the dental floss holder back into the deep recesses of the mouth.
3. Ask the client to hold this position and make sound. Do not tell him to say R. You want him to hold his position and produce sound. A good R may result.
4. If a good R sound results, repeat several times to solidify the position in the clients mind. Most clients will not tolerate the floss holder in the mouth too long without gagging. Clients usually gag less if they have control of the holder themselves. Let them hold it as they engage in this activity.
5. If a good sound can be practiced with the floss holder, the next step is to fade the use of the holder. As such, ask the client to try the position and produce the sound without the floss holder between trials. In other words, alternate between productions made with the floss holder and those without. See if you can establish the good sound without it. Once the Tip R begins to emerge, continue to use the dental floss holder as a guide whenever you need to restimulate the Tip R position. Also keep it on hand to warm up the tongue at the beginning of sessions. Use

the dental floss holder to continue increasing strength in the tongue as therapy progresses.

Some clients are able to curl the tip around the floss but are unable to pull the floss holder back into the oral cavity. If so, spend several weeks on this activity until enough strength is acquired to pull it in. Assign use of the dental floss holder as homework to exercise the tongue for the Tip R. Let the client take the holder home. Ask him to practice exercise curls a certain number of times every day. I usually ask clients to keep the floss holder in the bathroom with their toothbrush. I ask them to do ten curls every time they brush their teeth. This way, most kids practice ten times once or twice per day between therapy sessions. It usually takes a client less than thirty seconds to do this daily homework. Explain that to the client.

The client with an isolated R problem usually will learn a Tip R within a few weeks of its use if he is curling the tongue correctly. Readers are asked to obtain a dental floss holder and to engage in these procedures themselves in order to understand the method fully. Use one floss holder per client, and use new floss each session. And consider using two holders per client: one at home for practice and one in the office for direct instruction. Or have the client take it back and forth from home and therapy in a sandwich bag.

Adjust Jaw Position for Accurate Sound

In addition to the techniques offered above, the jaw and its movements must be addressed in most clients. Sometimes jaw movements need to be fixed before tongue work can be useful for R. Other times, a jaw position has to be adjusted to obtain a better acoustic quality. In either case, jaw facilitation techniques will need to be included.

How do we begin to address jaw position in Tip R therapy? In simple cases, we ask the client to move the jaw up or down slightly as the tongue adjusts to new positions. In these activities, we discover that some R sounds change radically with even slight adjustments to jaw position. The sound can snap into position suddenly as jaw position is altered. These clients can be asked to "bring up your jaw" or "lower your jaw a little bit."

Other clients have such poor awareness of their own oral mechanisms that we first have to teach them about the jaw and its movements before we can ask for adjustments. We also may have to give the client a tool with which to position the jaw correctly. The following ideas are are presented in no particular order.

- *Discover the Jaw:* Teach the client he has a jaw by talking about it, looking at the jaw in the mirror, feeling it, tapping it, vibrating it, watching chewing motions in a mirror, or looking at a picture of a skull to see the jawbone. Talk about bones and muscles, and teach the client that the jaw is a bone.
- *Discover Jaw Movement:* Help the client discover the jaw's movements by opening and closing the mouth, moving the jaw from side to side, and chewing in a mirror. Use dry snacks, chewy treats or gum. Have the client hold his jaw with his hands while performing these actions.

- *Stabilize the Jaw for a Wide Open Oral Position:* Help the client differentiate his tongue movements from those of the jaw by stabilizing the jaw with the mouth open wide during tongue exercises. Prop the mouth wide open by placing the side of a tongue depressor between the molars on one side of the mouth.
- *Stabilize the Jaw for a Narrow Open Oral Position:* Help the client stabilize the jaw with the mouth in a partially open position for rehearsal of R. Do so by having him bite onto a thin object at the molars. For example, use a baby tongue depressor, the stick of a Toothette®, the stick of an OraSwab®, a straw or coffee stir, a Bitestix® or the handle of a Nuk Oral Massager®. Begin with wider objects and move toward thin objects. Work on tongue position for R while the jaw is stabilized this way.
- *Increase Jaw Strength and Stability:* The easiest and most effective way to facilitate better jaw movement and stability for R is to facilitate better *clenching*. The clench of the jaw is an extra tight closure of the articulated teeth during biting or chewing. When clients practice the clench, they learn about and strengthen the biggest muscles that stabilize jaw movements for speech—the masseters. Have the client palpate the masseter muscles with his fingers while he clenches. Most R clients will be able to clench on demand like this, but a few will need to bite on a rubbery object to get the idea. Ask the client to count to ten or recite the alphabet while clenching to increase duration for the clenching action. Do *not* utilize this activity when cross bite or temporomandibular pain is present.

Use the Lips to Facilitate Tongue Position

Lip position has a strong influence on tongue position because of the close structural and neurological relationship between the two. Better tongue movement often can be facilitated by manipulating the movements and positions of the lips. This is easy to see when stimulating a Tip R position. The backward curl of the tongue tip for a Tip R can be facilitated by asking the client to retract the lips into a broad smile. The smiling position may distort the sound or may make it sound better. In either case, the back and lateral pull of the lips into a broad smile can cause the tongue tip to pull back further with more tension. In fact, some difficult clients are unable to get the tongue tip to sweep up and back unless they smile simultaneously. Use the smile liberally at first to help get the tip into position.

Retracting the lips while curling the tongue tip is a coordinated pattern that helps tongue tip position, but it is a pattern that cannot remain throughout an entire R program. We do not normally say R with that much lip retraction. Thus, the pattern will have to be broken up at some point. Ask the client to retract the lips while curling the tongue tip, and then to hold tongue position while bringing the lips forward. Most clients will lose good tongue position during this exercise but will learn the pattern over time.

Many clients can alter lip position simply by following a simple instruction like, "Poke your lips out," or, "Smile a little bit." But some clients cannot. Sometimes we first must teach our client that he has lips and can move them. The following ideas are offered in no particular order:

- *Discover the Lips:* Teach the client he has lips. Talk about them, look at them in the mirror, feel them, look at pictures of faces to see the lips, tap on the lips, vibrate them, move them around, put lip gloss or lipstick on them, or feel cold food or objects with them.
- *Discover Lip Movement:* Help the client discover lip movement. Have him open and close the mouth, pucker and retract the lips, pretend to kiss, and so forth. Also practice lip sounds like B, M, W and P. Have your client watch his lips in a mirror during these activities.
- *Activate the Lips:* Help the client's lip muscles to activate by stretching, vibrating, and pressing on them. Have him watch in a mirror for more feedback.

Getting the Lips Out of the Way

Some clients cannot produce a good Tip R sound because they cannot stop puckering during tongue movement. In this case, we have to use a mechanical means to get the lips out of the way. The easiest tool to use in this regard is the *lip retractor*.

The lip retractor is a device designed for use by orthodontists for photographing the teeth. Placed correctly in the mouth, the lip retractor pulls the lips laterally. With the lip retractor in place, most R clients will be unable to move the lips at all. This is a great way to help them focus on what their tongues should be doing. Put lip retractors in and have the client watch himself in a mirror. Most clients think that retractors are pretty cool. It gives them a scary look. So give the client a few minutes to look all around his mouth before he is required to work on his tongue. Lip retractors can get uncomfortable after a few moments, so allow the client to pull them out as needed. Encourage the client to keep his retractor in for increasing lengths of time so that he can do his tongue work. If possible, send a lip retractor home for additional practice.

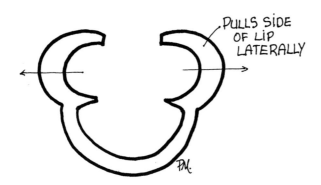

Fig. 7.6. The sides of the lip retractor can be held by the lateral margins of the lips. They push the lips away from midline to expose the teeth.

Combining Tip R with Back R Work

Some clients can learn an R only when Tip R methods are combined with Back R methods. Together, all these methods function to mature the tongue's movements to a point where a correct R can be produced. If you have tried all the methods of this chapter to no avail, begin to incorporate those of the next chapter. Consider integrating both types of methods when you start with clients.

Watch Tip-R Change to Back-R

One of the reasons the Back R is a more sophisticated and mature movement pattern for production of R is the simple fact that, given time and maturity, the Tip R often will change into a Back R. Clients who leave treatment having learned a Tip R often return for follow-up visits months or years later using a Back R. In the ensuing time after treatment ended, their oral movement skills for R continued to mature. This is a common phenomenon. The opposite—a Back R evolving into a Tip R—almost never occurs.

A standard principle of movement may explain this phenomenon. That is, all movements are based upon economy. The more economical a movement is, the more likely it is that it will be included in the body's repertoire of habits. A tongue tip that pulls far back toward the velum takes the tongue away from its neutral position. Tip retraction slows the tongue's movements and makes for more difficult transitions between R and other phonemes. Given the choice, the tongue will opt to stay closer to its neutral position. Remember, the Tip R and the Back R both include high elevation of the tongue's lateral margins for achieving their acoustic result. Thus, as tongue movement patterns for R mature, the tip extension to the rear will begin to fade away, and the high elevation of the tongue's lateral margins will remain. The sides will get stronger over time and dominate tongue position while tip retraction will become irrelevant to the overall sound of R. Thus, what began as a Tip R sound often transforms into a Back R.

Keep in mind that this phenomenon does not occur in all clients. The Tip R position can and does remain the production movement of choice for many of our clients, just as it does in the normal population. Further, some clients develop the habit over time of utilizing both the Tip R and Back R positions, depending upon word position and the coarticulatory effects of nearby phonemes.

~ Summary ~

- The heart of successful R therapy consists of a client's ability to position the jaw, lips and tongue in ways that will allow for the correct acoustic quality of R to result.

- The essential tongue movement needed for production of the Tip R is a sweeping up and back of the tongue tip so that it curls and approaches but does not touch the velum. This is called the *grand sweep*.

- The Tip R can be trained using a live visual model or a hand model to demonstrate the grand sweeping motion of the tongue tip.

- Clients can tap from L back along the palate until they reach position for a Tip R.

- Clients can slide from L to R or from Z to R to achieve correct tongue position for a Tip R.

- An external touch cue can be given to the back of the head in order to help clients learn to point and press the tongue tip in that direction for a Tip R.

- A dental floss holder is an excellent tool to guide and thin the tongue for the Tip R position. It is an excellent tool for resistance training when exercising the curling movement, and it will help increase overall tension in the tongue.

- Jaw and lip position can be altered intermittently during work to facilitate correct tongue position for R and in order to achieve the correct acoustic quality for R.

- Some clients can learn an R only when Tip R methods are combined with Back R methods.

- The Tip R often changes into a Back R over time. This reflects the body's natural tendency to resort to movements that are most efficient.

- The Tip R that is achieved as a result of these techniques is called the *cornerstone sound*. Production of the cornerstone sound marks the end of one phase of treatment and the beginning of another.

#8 Positioning the Tongue for a Back R
How to Attain a Nearly Impossible Position

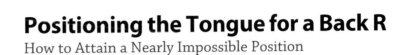

Many speech and language pathologists prefer to teach the Back R in therapy because it keeps the tongue closer to the neutral position for execution of R in complicated words and rapid conversational speech. The beautiful Back R can be the ticket out of therapy for "easy" clients, but it also can be the reason for failure in "hard" ones. Clients who cannot learn the tongue movements necessary for a Back R when that is the only R being addressed will experience failure no matter how long they are in treatment.

The Back R has several problems that make it more difficult to train than a Tip R. First, the Back R is hard to see. The essential movements are made in the deep recesses of the oral cavity. Clients can't see how to move the tongue, and therapists have trouble determining if their clients are moving the right way. Even when we shine a flashlight into the mouth, the tongue movements of this sound are too subtle. Thus, more verbal description of movement must be used. And although verbal description helps, the Back R can be hard to describe. This is especially true if the essential Back R movements are not understood well by the treating therapist.

In addition, Back R is difficult because it requires the use of the most mature tongue-movement patterns, which many clients have not, or cannot, learn. These movements are complicated. In fact, readers who have skipped ahead to this chapter for immediate treatment recommendations should first read the earlier chapters that describe the Back R in detail.

As we have described earlier, Back R is made by stabilizing the tongue at its back-lateral margins while the middle-back tenses forward into a slightly high position, and the lips round. The greatest mistake therapists make when facilitating the Back R is to ignore the movement difference between the tongue's back-lateral margins and its middle back. Failure occurs when clients are told simply to "lift the back." While this may assist the easiest of clients, it is too general for our difficult ones. The essence of a good Back R production rests in the client's ability to use the lateral backs as points of stability while differentially lifting and tensing the middle back.

Facilitation of tongue position for the Back R is achieved through visual, tactile and proprioceptive means. In general, methods should progress from simple gross-stimulation to complex refined input. The methods of this chapter are designed to elicit the client's first cornerstone sound through stimulation of the Back R. Please remember that each technique can be tried in one of four ways:

1. *Vocalic R Movements*. Produce a vowel first. Then glide into Back-R position.
2. *Consonantal R Movements*. Attain target position first. Voice at this apex. Continue to voice while gliding into a subsequent vowel.
3. *Isolated R Movements*. Move into target position in silence. Produce voice while in the apex position. Glide out of position in silence.
4. *Gross Sequences with R*: Babble with a big vowel ("Ah") and the Back R position. Go for gross approximations of the sound.

Verbal Description

Training the Back R almost always begins with a simple verbal description, such as "lift up the back of your tongue." Easy clients actually can learn to produce the Back R with this instruction alone. Remember, we begin with simple input and progress to more difficult and invasive procedures, so that we are never doing more than we have to. This saves time, money and energy, and it prevents us from encroaching on our clients when we don't have to. If a client can learn a Back R with this plain and unadorned direction, use it, accept it and rehearse it. The client has shown you that his basic oral-motor skills are good. He already knows how to use the back-lateral margins of the tongue naturally. Consider yourself lucky. Treat the response as the client's cornerstone sound and drill it until he can produce it spontaneously. Then move on. If you have not been quite this fortunate, however, provide additional input.

The Live Visual Model

The live visual model also can be effective in teaching the Back R to clients with good oral-motor development. When we model the Back R, we usually do so with exaggeration, to make the sound easier to see. Remember, the Back R by itself is nearly impossible to view because the mouth is only partially open and the essential tongue movements are made in the back. To model the Back R so clients have a slight chance to see it, open the mouth very wide.

Try opening your mouth as wide as it will go and producing a Back R sound. Retract the lips to get them completely out of the way. The reader will realize immediately that R distorts somewhat when the mouth is open that far. Therapists must experiment with the degree of their own mouth opening to find the position in which the mouth is open far enough for easy interoral viewing but not too far that the sound is distorted. Also, therapists should practice this method on their own until they *can* produce an excellent R with the mouth fully open. Visual inspection during this modeled production usually reveals a tongue that is retracted and humping up toward the velum with the sides slightly higher than the middle, yet the middle is high too. That's okay. Despite the fact that a true Back R is made with differential control of the lateral backs and the middle back, simply knowing that the sound is made in the back is enough for many clients to learn the sound.

Clients who can learn a Back R sound from this gross visual model can apply their habitually correct pattern to any new movement. An excellent R sound results. If an adequate R sound results, celebrate! Then rehearse it and prepare to move on to more advanced stages of the program.

The Puppet or Hand Model
A puppet or hand model can be used early in treatment to teach gross upward elevation of the back of the tongue for production of the Back R. But they do not demonstrate the differential control needed in the back. Hand and puppet models can be effective for those clients with adequate oral-motor skills, just like the live visual model. The following are recommended when using a hand model—a bare hand, a puppet with a tongue that can house a hand, or a sock on the hand.

1. Ask the client to pretend that your hand is a tongue. Explain that the fingertips will be the tongue tip, and the wrist area will be the back of the tongue.
2. Hold the hand flat with the palm down and the fingertips facing the client. Move the wrist up and down to simulate the up-and-down movement of the back of the tongue.
3. Use your other hand to hold the fingertips still so the client can see that the tongue tip remains down.
4. Produce a Back R with your mouth as you model it with your hand. Make sure that the up-and-down movements of your wrist coincide with those of your tongue back.

If an adequate R sound is the result of this gross modeling, accept it, celebrate it, rehearse it, and prepare to move on to advanced stages of the program. If a correct R sound cannot be achieved with a hand or puppet model, move on to new and different stimuli.

Schematic Illustrations
Schematic illustrations allow the trainer to teach the Back R in a gross fashion. They also allow a therapist to go into more detail about the differential use of the middle and lateral backs. Schematic illustrations are offered throughout this chapter.

The Essential Butterfly Position
The *butterfly position* is a systematic way to teach differential control of the lateral backs from the middle back. It can be used to teach the isolated apex-R position. There are four basic steps one uses to achieve the butterfly position: bite, push, slide and voice. Each step is described in detail below. They are a little tricky. Readers are strongly urged to learn each step by themselves before using them with clients. We have broken down the movements of the Back R into four parts. These details can be difficult to grasp at first. Do not fret if you cannot do each step on first trial. Allow yourself several days, weeks or months to understand this material and to perform these actions well. Even if you already can produce a perfect Back R yourself, you may find these directions hard to follow. Read them slowly.

Let the ideas sink in as you try the actions. Review this material periodically until you have a thorough understanding of the actions involved. And practice with another therapist who does know how the butterfly position works.

STEP 1: BITE

1. Draw the client's attention to the back-lateral margins of the tongue through visual and tactile means. Brush or rub the back-lateral margins with a tool of semi-rough texture. A toothbrush, Nuk® massager, Toothette®, or OraSwab® work well. Brush back and forth two or three times on each side. Watch in a mirror, and use a schematic illustration of the tongue to highlight the lateral margins. Draw arrows to illustrate the brushing action there. Use explicit labels like "the sides of the tongue" or "the back on the sides." Make sure your client knows where the lateral margins of the tongue are.

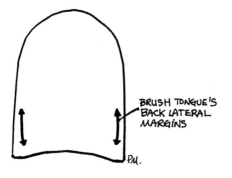

Fig. 8.1. Brush the lateral margins of the tongue to increase general tactile awareness of these areas.

2. Ask the client to bite the back-lateral margins of the tongue with the upper and lower molars. Have him do so gently but firmly. The molars are located almost immediately above and below the back-lateral margins, so most clients will not have difficulty with this.
3. Some clients will be able to bite down on the back-lateral margins right away. If so, move on to Step Two below. If not, assign step number one above as homework to be done in conjunction with daily tooth brushing. Ask the client to brush the sides of the tongue at the back once or twice a day after brushing his teeth. Ask him to brush back and forth four times on each side. Even if the client brushes his tongue only two or three times during the week, his awareness of the back-lateral margins will improve significantly by the time he returns to the next session.

STEP 2: PUSH

1. After the client can bite down on the back-lateral margins, ask him to push the back-lateral margins of the tongue upward against the upper molars. It should feel like he is pressing against the molars with the sides of the back of his tongue. The client should push with both sides simultaneously. This action will teach the client to elevate the lateral margins upward quite high. Eventually, the client will not need

lateral elevation this high to produce a good R, but he needs it now to learn the essential position.

2. Once the client begins to push the back-lateral margins of the tongue upward against the upper molars, ask him next to open the mouth wide by lowering the jaw and spreading the lips. This way the lateral margins of the tongue will stretch very high.
3. Visual inspection of this position from the front should reveal that the tongue is high on the sides and low in the middle. This is the basic butterfly position. It also could be described with other metaphors, such as *hills* on the sides with a *valley* in the middle.

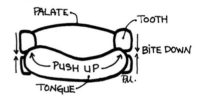

Fig. 8.2. The butterfly position from the front. Note that the sides are high and the middle is depressed.

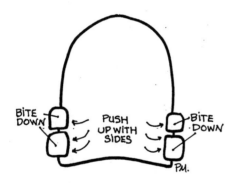

Fig. 8.3. The butterfly position from the top. Note that the sides are high and the middle is depressed.

4. Ask the client to hold this position. Repeat several times to rehearse the movement in silence. Use the mirror to help the client see what he has achieved. Reward him for achieving this position. Half of his work is done.
5. Assign the butterfly position as homework for the week. Even if his position is weak and poorly executed, it makes for a good home practice routine. Ask the client to practice it three times every evening when he brushes his teeth. Challenge him to see if he can conquer this action. If he practices through the week, he will return with a significantly improved butterfly position. Once the butterfly is strong and dependable, you may move on to step 3.

STEP 3: SLIDE

The position achieved through steps one and two above bring the sides of the tongue up, but the position usually is too far forward to achieve an acoustically correct R. Now the tongue has to be brought further back into the oral cavity. As such, teach the client to slide the basic butterfly position back further into the mouth. This can be done in two basic ways.

1. *Slide the Butterfly Back*: Ask the client to hold the butterfly position firm and then to slide the whole tongue further back toward the oropharynx. "Don't let your tongue come out of the butterfly position. Slide it back along the molars so that you feel the sides of your tongue scraping against the bottom of your top molars. Keep the sides high while you are moving the tongue back." If the client can perform this action correctly, move on to "Step 4: Voice."
2. *Incorporate Tip Curling*: The second way we can bring the butterfly position further back into the oral cavity is to have the client curl the tip back while holding the butterfly position. This is like holding the butterfly position while performing a Tip R. Curling the tip will help slide the entire tongue back. If he keeps the sides high, a great Back R should result. If the client has had no prior experience with the Tip R, take a few minutes to teach the curling position all by itself. You may find that the client can achieve a good R sound with the Tip R alone. If so, use common sense and immediately drop your work on the Back R and switch your training to the Tip R!
3. *Combine 1 and 2*. Many clients can achieve good position when the above techniques above are combined or alternated. Some clients can attain a good R sound within one session this way. Others will have to combine or alternate these practice routines many times over for many weeks before they achieve a good R sound.

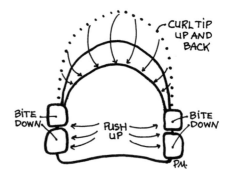

Fig. 8.4. Combine the actions of the Back R with those of the Tip R to achieve correct oral position.

STEP 4: VOICE

Check each tongue position throughout this process by asking the client to voice while the position is held. Never ask him to say R or he will switch back to his habitual incorrect position. Remember, you are not training the sound; you are training the *position*. Don't worry about what the resultant phoneme sounds like along the way. And avoid showing disappointment when the client does not make a good R. At some point in this process, a good R will result when tongue position is just right. Celebrate as soon as you hear it. In the meantime, give other words of encouragement and instruction. "Perfect. It does not sound like R yet, but you did exactly what I told you to do."

Once an R of good quality is heard, prepare to help the client stabilize this position with drill. This is his cornerstone R, so don't let it go if at all possible. Then get ready to move on to more advanced stages of the program.

Some clients will fail miserably throughout these exercises because these movements are difficult to conceptualize and carry out. They will need further work to organize tongue movements. Usually, this work is a replaying of all the techniques described so far while working on other aspects of the program. Rotate all these techniques in and out of your sessions until that point of magic is reached and a perfect R is produced. Seriously consider switching to a Tip R if the client seems impaired in making tongue movements according to the directions in this section. Or alternate your stimulation between Tip R and the Back R to develop tongue mobility and control. This work will reveal the type of R for which the client will eventually be suitable. Consider teaching a W-for-R substitution in lieu of the good R that will emerge later. And focus considerable time on training his mouth to switch rapidly from the other three glides—W, L and Y.

The External Tactile Cue

An *external tactile cue* on the head can be used to teach tongue position for the Back R like it did for a Tip R. Remember, an external tactile cue entails the use of touch on the outside of the head to instruct or remind a client about tongue movement. The external cue for the Back R is a nice supplement to the methods described above, but it rarely works as a sole technique. In other words, the external cue can be effective once the tongue has been explored by other visual, verbal and tactile means.

Since the primary action of the Back R consists of lifting the back-lateral margins, the external tactile cue for the Back R is given to points on either side of the head. Use your fingers to press against both sides of the head simultaneously, pointing toward where the lateral margins extend. Ask the client to "push the sides of your tongue toward my fingers." Each client will require a slightly different position, so experiment with them—above the ears, at the temporomandibular joints, at the temples, on the top of the head. Even points on the jaw or the lower molars can work at times.

Use the client's production of sound to test the effectiveness of your finger positioning. Try one position and ask for sound. Then move your fingers to a slightly different position and ask for more sound. Sometimes the oddest position will stimulate a correct R sound. A good R sound will result if position is correct and enough tension is generated. If so, reward and rehearse this cornerstone sound. If a good R sound does not result, change the position of your fingers on the head. Also, combine the external tactile cues of the Tip R with those of the Back R to bring these two movement patterns together.

The Internal Tactile Cue

An *internal tactile cue* is a hint given by an object directly to the tongue to facilitate appropriate movement. As we have stated, the essential movement to be facilitated for a Back R is upward lateral extension of the tongue's back-lateral margins. To use an internal tactile cue, we place an object between the back molars on both sides. The client reaches toward and pushes against these objects with the back sides of the tongue.

Ask your client to chew and soften a stick of gum. Then ask him to break the wad in half and place one piece between the upper and lower molars on one side, and the same on the other. The wads of gum will be positioned perfectly for the client to learn which part of the tongue to push and in which direction. Ask the client to produce sound while pushing laterally against the gum wads. Ask him to push hard to increase tension throughout the back of the tongue.

If your client cannot manage the wads of gum, consider using an item with a handle. For example, use Toothettes®. Place the sponge ends of two Toothettes between the molars on both sides of the mouth simultaneously. Ask the client to reach for the sponges with the sides of his tongue in the same way that he reached for the wads of gum.

Adjusting Jaw Position for Accurate Sound
Working with the mouth wide open helps us put maximum attention on the tongue, and it helps the tongue learn to move independently from the jaw. But a good R, especially a good Back R, cannot be made by our clients when their mouths are wide open. Therefore, the jaw must be adjusted upward after the tongue has begun to move in a correct back position. Experiment with the level of jaw elevation to discover the position that facilitates the best Back R sound. Once you discover it, draw the client's attention to it visually and verbally. Help him stabilize it. Employ objects upon which the client can bite to stabilize the mouth in a partially open position. For example, have the client bite on a tongue depressor, Bitestix®, baby tongue depressor, straw, or coffee stirrer, or the handles of a Toothette®, OroSwab®, or swizzle stick.

Positioning the Lips to Influence the Tongue
Many clients can be helped in tongue position for a Back R by positioning the lips into a more posterior and retracted position. Ask the client to smile broadly and tightly as he elevates the lateral backs of the tongue. Retracted tension in the lips can generalize to the tongue and help it generate more overall tension and lift the sides. Once the correct acoustic quality for R is attained, the lips can be taught to relax and round to create an even better sound.

Getting the Lips Out of the Way
Some clients cannot produce a good Back R sound because they cannot stop puckering the lips during tongue movement practice. In this case, too, we have to use a mechanical means to get the lips out of the way. The easiest tool to use in this regard is the lip retractor.

With the lip retractor in place, most R clients will be unable to move the lips at all. This is a great way to help them focus on what their tongues should be doing. Encourage the client to keep his retractor in for increasing lengths of time so that he can keep it in while he does his tongue work. Send a lip retractor home for practice.

Adjusting Lip Position for Accurate Sound
Once the tongue has begun to achieve an adequate position for the Back R, lip position can be adjusted to fine tune the acoustic quality of the sound. A truly good Back R sound usually has some amount of lip rounding. The client must be asked to hold his tongue in the retracted position while rounding the lips slightly. This can be difficult for some clients because it requires diametrically opposed actions—pulling the tongue back while rounding the lips forward. The forward movement of the lips often triggers anterior movement of the tongue that breaks up the posterior position just learned. The client may need several sessions on lip movements to help him differentiate their movements from those of the tongue.

The amount of lip rounding needed for a correct Back R sound can vary tremendously from one client to another. Some clients even can make a Back R with no lip rounding at all. Various lip positions must be tried in order to discover the lip position that renders the best Back R sound for each individual client.

— Summary —

- Many speech and language pathologists prefer to teach the Back R. It keeps the tongue closer to the neutral position for execution of R in rapid conversational speech.

- The Back R is hard to see, cumbersome to describe and difficult to facilitate. It requires the use of the most mature movement patterns of which the tongue is capable in speech.

- Back R is made by stabilizing the tongue at its back-lateral margins while the middle back tenses forward into a slightly high position that is lower than the sides, and the lips round.

- Training the Back R almost always begins with a simple verbal description, "Lift up the back of your tongue." Some clients can learn to produce the Back R with this unadorned instruction because their overall oral-motor development is good and they already use the back-lateral margins for stability in all speech movements.

- The live visual model can be quite effective as a beginning technique to teach the Back R in those clients with good oral-motor development.

- A hand or puppet model is a simple method for teaching gross upward elevation of the back of the tongue for production of the Back R. A tongue puppet can be quite effective for those clients with adequate oral-motor skills.

- Schematic illustrations allow the trainer to teach the Back R in a gross fashion or to go into more detail about the use of the middle and lateral backs.

- The butterfly position is a way to teach clients to elevate the sides and depress the middle of the tongue for production of a Back R.

- An external tactile cue is given to the sides of the head and toward which the lateral margins extend for a Back R. An external cue for a Back R can be used in combination with those used for the Tip R.

- Experiment with the level of jaw elevation to discover the position that facilitates the best Back R sound possible. Clients can bite on objects to stabilize the mouth in a partially open position.

- A retracted lip position can facilitate better tongue position while learning the Back R.

- A lip retractor pulls the lips out of the way for work on the Back R.

- Lip position is adjusted to fine tune the acoustic quality of the Back R sound. Level of lip rounding necessary differs between clients.

- Some clients can learn an R only when the Back R methods of this chapter are combined with the Tip R methods of the prior chapter.

- The Back R that is achieved as a result of these techniques is called the *cornerstone sound*. Production of the cornerstone sound marks the end of one phase of treatment and the beginning of another.

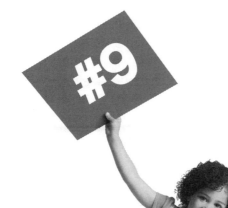

#9 Locking in on the Cornerstone R
Assure Success with a Solid Foundation

In the two prior chapters we learned methods to facilitate a client's first correct R sound, the production we have called his *cornerstone sound*. The cornerstone sound could be a Tip R or a Back R, and it could be a Vocalic R, Consonantal R or an R embedded in a vowel or consonant sequence. Once produced, an easy client can begin to repeat his cornerstone sound within a few minutes. When old enough to understand what he is doing, the easy client can begin to use this new sound in the production of all kinds of words. He may do so clumsily, but he will do so almost immediately. The easy adolescent or adult client will begin to think about all the words containing R that have plagued him throughout the years, and he will try to say them correctly during that first session. We usually have to slow these clients down as they zoom forward into difficult words that are beyond their immediate capacity.

Easy clients can generalize production of R to all phonetic contexts with ease. On rare occasions, an exceptional client can learn his cornerstone R during one session and return to the next session with near perfect mastery in conversational speech. Parents and teachers always praise us for the easy client's astounding and rapid success. We should not deter them from these compliments, of course, but we should realize that technique is only a small part of what moved him forward so fast. It was his natural ability that allowed easy sound acquisition. A client who progresses this fast has outstanding auditory skills, and his oral-motor skills are fully mature. This client only needs straightforward information about how to position the mouth, especially the tongue, for R. Sometimes, it's a wonder that exceptionally easy clients need therapy in the first place.

The difficult client is another story. Once he has learned a basic cornerstone sound, the difficult client needs to be led step by painful step from his initial cornerstone sound to completion of the program. This process can be so slow that it can seem as if the client has reached a plateau. Carryover to conversational speech of the client's limited skills will be nil. Stagnation and an apparent inability to complete the program will seem like failure to the client, parents and therapist. Treatment like this can drag on for years. When I am referred these difficult clients, the referring therapist usually reports, "He can say R, sort of, on some words. But he just doesn't get it. We've been doing the same thing for years. I don't know what else to do to help him." Hopelessness can set in.

Stagnation is not failure.

A client who is stuck needs careful assistance to take him through the stages of R maturation. He has gained some initial skill. Now he needs to learn to take that skill into more difficult speech tasks by working in small carefully determined steps. These tiny divisions of treatment are unnecessary for the easy client, but they can be the only means of success for the difficult one.

The biggest mistake that most therapists make to cause their clients to get stuck in therapy is to assume that the client is ready to produce a variety of words with R right after he has learned to say his cornerstone R. This is not a good plan for difficult cases. A tough client cannot generalize the R sound he has learned for his cornerstone R to any other phonetic environments. Depressed levels of auditory discrimination and poor oral-motor control have caused trouble learning to say R in the first place. Now these problems plague him as he uses his new R in the sophisticated movement patterns of words. The difficult client will not succeed when we simply *hope* that he will improve with enough practice on a wide variety of R words. The opposite is true: Working on a wide variety of R words can be the primary cause of stagnation.

Every word that contains an R is comprised of its own unique environment of vowels and consonants. Consider the phonetic environment of two words: *are* and *squirrel*. These words are complete opposites in terms of the complexity of oral movement they demand. The phonetic environment and the oral movements required for *are* are so simple that this sequence can qualify as a cornerstone sound for many clients. On the other hand, the phonetic environment of the word *squirrel* is so complex that it almost always is one of the last R words a client conquers. Using a word list that uses these and other words of uncontrolled phonetic environments is a disservice to the difficult client. It requires the client to take immediate control of his newly learned skill. It's like asking a beginning gymnast who has just learned a cartwheel on a mat to perform it on a 4-inch balance beam. Although the basic skill has emerged, the requirements of the advanced task are too difficult and too early in the training program.

Every word is comprised of its own unique series of consonants and vowels. The oral movements required to move into and away from R depend upon that word's phonetic environment. The difficult client needs to learn to on-glide and off-glide around his new R sound from a variety of positions—the *transition skills*. Transition work is the oral-motor need after the cornerstone R has emerged. Transition work will be the essence of the rest of the client's therapy. He will need to get unstuck in small, carefully chosen steps based upon the coarticulatory environment of the R phoneme.

Successful R therapy for seemingly hopeless clients requires the artful application of selected methods to move oral-motor transition skills forward. We are in a contest with the misarticulated R. Victory requires the application of brilliant tactics that draw the client forward from the isolated production of a cornerstone R sound to the ability to use a correct R freely in rapid and unmonitored conversational speech.

The key to building a successful R program for difficult clients is to identify the cornerstone sound, use it as the base of operation, and move cautiously from there. This is a gradual modification of the cornerstone R. If correct, this sound can be the basis for the client's entire treatment program. This is called an *idiosyncratic hierarchy of R therapy based on a cornerstone sound*, a regimented approach to articulation therapy that is much more stringent than that proposed by our early teachers. This approach is not represented in common workbooks for R therapy.

This chapter reflects the most exacting of all plans that will be necessary for the most difficult R clients. The wise therapist, of course, will recognize how this hierarchy must be altered for individual clients. She will see that easy clients can be trained in this way in just a few lessons. We begin this chapter with the therapist's immediate response to the cornerstone sound, and we end it with the client speaking the cornerstone R correctly in structured conversational games. Later chapters will review techniques to help the client break away from his reliance on the cornerstone sound and to branch into all phonetic environments for R production.

Lock In on the Cornerstone R

No matter how the cornerstone R arrives, there it is! *Hooray*! As a speech and language pathologist, we usually greet this R as a small miracle. Don't be in a hurry. The sound may appear again, but the cornerstone R happens when all factors are right. The client may have no idea that he said a good sound or how it occurred. It's like the first time a baby says *momma*. Just because he said it once does not ensure he will say it again any time soon. What should we do?

- Once we hear the cornerstone sound, our goal must be to acknowledge the sound. A simple "Yes!" lets the client know you are pleased with the sound he produced.
- The most important thing to do with the cornerstone sound is to get the client to repeat it. If the client said it once, have him do it twice, and if he says it twice, have him do it three times, and so forth. We want to lock in on that first sound. Don't try to be fancy with this work. Simply say, "That's it. Say it again. . . . Say it again. . . . Again. . . . Once more." Try not to let the sound get away once it appears.
- Keep all other distractions away. Don't let the client take a turn in a game. Don't talk to him about how it feels to make the sound. And don't get up to get him a reward. Don't even make a big deal of it. Do nothing to distract him from the tactile, proprioceptive and auditory sensation he just had. You want him to sense it again and again if possible.
- If the client cannot repeat the sound immediately, try one or two more times and then drop it. Do not beat it into the ground. Retreat to your stimulation techniques.
- Do not show disappointment if the client loses the sound during these early sessions. You do not want him to think he has failed you. The opposite is true: He has just demonstrated a tiny piece of success. Celebrate that. "Alright! You did it. I heard one perfect one today. We are on our way."

- End the work on R right then, or switch topics and focus on something else. Get the client's mind off the work for a few minutes. Have a little conversation about something of interest to give his brain a rest. The client has made a neurological connection that will appear again if you don't force it before he is ready.
- After a break, try again. If he can do it again, rehearse it. If not, let it go for the time being. Again, reward him for the tiny piece of success he has achieved.

After the session, think through the work. Were there any connections between your stimulation and the client's correct response? Often, the correct R arrives after the avenues of treatment converge. It may not have been one specific technique that caused this sound to emerge; it may have been the combination of several. The cornerstone R may have arrived as planned or it may have shown up as a complete surprise. What matters is that the sound was attained. With this emergence comes a responsibility to study the process and determine what has contributed to its arrival. This mental work on your part will greatly enhance the client's ability to perform well in subsequent sessions. It also will help you with succeeding clients.

Use the Cornerstone R

Now we know there are ways to get him to say a correct R sound. The goal of each of the next few sessions should be to reach that point again without assuming that it will occur. I often ask the client in the next session if he remembers what we did the last time. Then I ask him to say R again just as he did before. Some clients were so excited to learn R in the previous session that they have practiced it correctly all week. Other clients remember having learned a good R and have rehearsed it all week, but they have been practicing it wrong because their skill deteriorated right after they left the treatment room. Still, others do not even remember what they did that morning, let alone what they learned the previous week. In any case, treatment must begin again. The client may take another few weeks to find it again, but don't worry. He is not failing; he is *learning*. Give him time. Revisit all the auditory, visual, tactile and proprioceptive stimulation techniques you have been using over the past several weeks. The client will find that unique sound again. After a while, he will make it consistently.

Once the sound reappears, don't change anything you are doing. Failure in therapy is almost assured for tough clients when we move too quickly away from this cornerstone sound. Don't think about other ways to make the sound. Don't bring out the word lists. Don't try to alter the vowel. Concentrate on repeating this cornerstone sound.

Help the Client Hear His Cornerstone Sound

Engage in activities to bring the cornerstone sound to the client's conscious awareness and to help him make its production consistent and automatic. Remember, just because a client can *produce* his first good R sound does not mean he can *hear* it. Drill on productions of this new sound and use this time to train his ear. It is far better for the client to repeat his cornerstone R sound fifty times while learning to discriminate it, than for him to move on to anything else. Think of it as one note on a piano keyboard that a piano tuner is adjusting.

The child must learn to strike the key in such a way that the right tone is achieved every time. Then he can incorporate that single note into slightly more complex movement tasks. Be systematic in your attempts to train the client's ear. Teach him to lock in on its acoustic qualities. This process can take weeks, or even months in some cases. The following ideas guide the process.

- Train the client to recognize the differences between his own good and bad productions by clearly judging the attempts for him. "Yes, that one was perfect. . . . No, that one was no good." Make clear distinctions between good and bad productions so the client can learn to produce the sound one way or the other. Use terms that are black and white. Avoid gray responses, like, "Okay, that was a good try." Wimpy feedback offers the client no information at all.
- Ask the client to produce a certain number of cornerstone R sounds clearly and steadily in a sequence. For example, challenge him to say ten in a row and to make each one exactly the same. Work slowly and carefully. Stop him immediately when his sound begins to wander and move toward the distortion category. Don't let him bend his sound.
- Focus the client's ear on his sound wandering. Use explicit terms to tune his ear. "The sound started to change. Did you hear it? You were going along and saying very good sounds, and then you started to lose it. Could you hear that?"
- As time passes, ask the client what happened to bend the sound. "Why did the sound change? What did you do differently to make the sound begin to change?"
- Help the client formulate his thoughts about his distorting sound by giving him words to describe the process. For example, the client might say his "mouth was going all weird." Put this in more explicit terms by saying, "Yes. I don't think you were getting the tip high enough."
- Test the client's ear periodically to see if he has begun to recognize his cornerstone R sound. "Was that correct?" You may be amazed at how often your client cannot make this simple distinction regarding his own productions. Continue to judge his productions for him as long as necessary. Begin to back off this feedback as the client's own ear improves and his responses to this question become consistently correct.

Introduce a Cornerstone Word

Easy clients can rehearse a random assortment of words once R begins to emerge. But the difficult R client needs to discover how to use his cornerstone R in specific words. Begin to do so by moving into a single word that perfectly reflects the cornerstone R motor pattern. This is the *cornerstone word*. Activate the client's listening skills and his powers of analysis by asking him if what he is saying sounds like anything familiar. Imitate his sound back to him exactly as he says it. Then ask, "Does it sound like any words you know?" Help him recognize that the sequence of sounds he is making sounds like a certain word. For example, say that your client has learned to say a vocalic Tip R after the vowel "Ah." He will be saying "Ah-R." Reveal to him that by saying "Ah-R" he actually is saying the word *are* with prolongation and exaggeration. Write the word in big block letters and say it several times. Point to each letter as you speak the unfolding word slowly. Have the client rehearse the word while pointing to the letters himself.

Good cornerstone words include *are, or, ear, rah, row, rye* and so forth. The most common cornerstone words are *are* and *rah*. The combination of R and Ah is the easiest for most clients. The wide open and low oral posture for Ah is a fantastic contrast with the high and tight oral posture for R. And these sounds have very different acoustic qualities.

Reward your client well for saying his cornerstone word correctly. After all, it's his first word with R! Encourage the client to say the cornerstone word exactly as he says his cornerstone sound. Do not worry if the word sounds odd because of its prolonged and exaggerated nature. Make absolutely sure that the apex R position is spoken perfectly. Rehearse this first word many times. Give the word a title, like "The Best Word" or "The First Correct Word." The production of this word is the client's first step on the path toward conversational speech. The cornerstone word should be rehearsed over time in such a way the client eventually is able to say it without much thought.

Practice Phrases, Sentences and Questions with the Cornerstone Word
The cornerstone word is the first and only oral-motor pattern the client has learned that incorporates his new acoustically correct R. Teach him to use it in gradually more difficult speech/motor tasks. First, move delicately by building other sounds and syllables around it. Keep the cornerstone word exactly as it is. Construct simple phrases, sentences and questions. Make sure to rehearse as slowly as the client needs for success so that the cornerstone word is uttered perfectly every time. Allow him to exaggerate the word in these grammatical constructions in the same way he did when he said it alone. Write each sample down in block letters for rehearsal. The following examples continue with our sample word *are*.

- Rehearse simple two-word utterances with the cornerstone word at the end: *You are. We are. They are. People are. Cats are. Dogs are.*
- Rehearse simple two-word utterances with the cornerstone word at the beginning: *Are we? Are they? Are walking. Are gone.*
- Rehearse simple three-word utterances with the cornerstone word at the end: *The boys are. The girls are. My cats are. Two dogs are.*
- Rehearse simple three-word utterances with this word at the beginning: *Are they gone? Are they fast? Are we in? Are you going?*
- Rehearse simple four- or five-word sentences with the cornerstone word embedded in the utterance: *The boys are here. My shoes are gone. The men are helping me. They are in the house.*

All this work should be done with perfect R sounds in perfect, cornerstone R words as the client has learned them to this point. Try to construct these practice phrases to be void of other R sounds, and simply ignore the few that may appear. Do not worry if the client has to slow down and exaggerate his cornerstone words in these tasks. Allow him to pause and regroup before and after each cornerstone word. Insist on accuracy. Add speed slowly, and only if it does not interfere with accuracy. In other words, sacrifice speed for accuracy during these early sessions.

Whatever the client has to do to say his cornerstone word perfectly, let him do those things. He is learning new oral-motor patterns, ones he has never done before. He needs to feel confident that he can take his time to do them well. These phrases and sentences make great homework practice if the client is performing well in therapy. Encourage the client to say these phrases and sentences the same way at home that he did in your room. Remind him to work slowly and to go for perfect R sounds all the time. Do not worry about how many different phrases, sentences or questions the client can say well. If he can say only one, highlight that one by rehearsing it many times in a variety of ways, and drop the rest.

Test Generalization Skills
It is tempting to assume that a client who has achieved the ability to practice words, phrases and sentences with a cornerstone R word is ready to generalize his new R into other phonetic contexts. It is tempting to move on to new words with R in new positions. Watch out! Most difficult clients are unable to do so. Spot test this ability to determine if there are any other patterns that can be added, but don't count on it. In most cases, we must stick with the cornerstone sound and word for a longer period of time before moving on to other contexts. Take baby steps as outlined below.

Add Phonetic Elements to the Cornerstone Word
Help your client continue to develop mastery over the cornerstone word by adding other sounds to it to create new words. If the client can say the cornerstone word *are*, add consonants to the beginning of this sound sequence to create *bar, jar, car* and so forth. Or add a phoneme to the end and rehearse *art, ark* and *arm*. The addition of these new phonemes creates a *basic word set* from which we can design many different practice lists. Rehearse all these basic words slowly and carefully so the integrity of the cornerstone sound is maintained throughout. And use the same cornerstone sound pattern over which he has control in slightly more complex phonetic combinations.

A cornerstone R that is produced in the vocalic position lends itself nicely to rhyming words when consonants are added to the beginning. For example, *bar, jar, far, car, star* and *czar* all rhyme with *are*. A Consonantal R does not lend itself to such rhyming. When a client has acquired the cornerstone sound Rah, words like *rock, rob, Ron* and *rot* must be used. These don't rhyme, but they contain the same cornerstone sound pattern in slightly more difficult oral-motor patterns.

Many clients have to learn these new patterns by separating the new consonants from the cornerstone sequence as they are spoken. For example, a student may say *bar* by pausing and regrouping after the B. This is just fine. We are giving the client every opportunity to speak these things correctly. Remember, we are not *testing* the client; we are *teaching* him.

Add Morphemic Elements to the Cornerstone Word
We can add even more challenging movements to the words in the basic word set by adding *morphemes* to them. The morpheme is the smallest unit of speech that has meaning. We can

add the plural morpheme to our practice words to produce the words *bars, jars, cars* and *stars*. We also can make our words more complex by adding whole syllables. For example, stretch *bar* into *barbell*, and *par* into *partake*.

Words of gradually increasing complexity can be practiced in sequence, such as: *mar, mark, market, marketplace, Marketplace Mall*. Allow the client whatever time he needs to make each sequence perfect. Ignore any other R's that may occur in the words. An interesting activity ensues when we create sequences that incorporate real and nonsense words. A list might be constructed with *car, card, cardoodle, cardoodlebug, cardoodlebugaronie!* The freedom to make up increasingly lengthy silly words makes therapy fun. It encourages kids to practice the same speech movement pattern over and over again without getting bored.

Rote Verbal Sequences with the Cornerstone Word

Once a client can produce one cornerstone word, it can be rehearsed in sequences as a way to move him toward conversational speech. If the client can say Ah-R and *are*, then he also can use this pattern to name the letter R. The name of the letter R can be one of his basic words. He can embed it into any combination that requires the use of that letter. For example, the client can recite the alphabet and embed that sound, "A, B, C, D, E, F, G, H, I, J, K, L, M, N, O, P, Q, Ah-R, S, T, U, V, W, X, Y, Z." This sequence can be repeated slowly to make sure the client says letter R correctly. It can be sung. And it can be repeated many times in a row. Additionally, the client might practice "Q, Ah-R, S" five times in a row.

Another way to embed letter R is to spell aloud a list of words that contain it. Continuing with our example, the client might spell *road* as "Ah-R, O, A, D." These simple routines ensure that the client rehearses his cornerstone sound or word in a conversational speech style before he is ready to tackle the demands of real conversation.

Counting also makes an excellent rote verbal sequence if the client has learned the R of the words *three* or *four*. For example, if the client can say a correct R in the number *four*, he could count through the forties: *forty, forty-one, forty-two, forty-three*, etc. Or he could make lists of other numbers that incorporate three or four: *twenty-four, thirty-four, forty-four*, etc. This is fantastic drill on the same oral-motor pattern. It is a skill that will have quick reward in the classroom or at home, and it is a wonderful step toward conversation.

Move into Conversational Games with the Cornerstone Word

The next step is to take the cornerstone word into conversational speech. This is a significant departure from traditional methods. Instead of holding conversation until the end of the program, we branch into conversation early in treatment so the client can learn to embed the oral-motor pattern he has just learned into his existing oral-motor patterns. Moving into conversation early also provides an opportunity for the client to think about this new movement as his mind stretches to include new ideas. However, you do not want to move into a general conversation. It probably would derail him at this early point with too many R words. Remember that your client has learned only one oral-movement pattern, cornerstone sound and cornerstone word. You must generate a speech event that resembles a conversation but is more controlled so it includes many instances of the cornerstone word.

One way to accomplish this is to play verbal games that incorporate the cornerstone word. For example, construct a guessing game with the sample word *are*. For his turn, have the client guess something about the therapist by incorporating *are* into his questions. Give answers that steer him toward the correct answer.

- The client can guess the therapist's age: "Are you 40? Are you 25? Are you 31?"
- The client can ask questions to determine what the therapist is planning for an upcoming break: "Are you going on vacation? Are you going to be working? Are you driving somewhere? Are you going to paint your house? Are you getting a puppy?"
- The client can ask the therapist her national background: "Are you Irish? Are you Jamaican? Are you Russian?"

You will have no control over the R sounds that will appear in these conversational games. Don't worry, and certainly don't correct them. In fact, instruct the client to ignore them. Tell him you do not care about the R sounds in any other words in these questions. Tell him to focus on and make perfect the cornerstone word. And continue to sacrifice speed for accuracy throughout this process.

The Speech Driving Range
Now we have moved our client quickly from production of the simple cornerstone sound to conversation. Notice, however, that the basic cornerstone sound has not changed throughout all the activities presented so far. The vowel has not changed, nor has the position of R in the syllable. In fact, the whole process has taken place with only one oral-motor pattern. This is a critical element of successful R therapy for the hard client, and it is a practice that has many advantages. First, keeping the cornerstone sound the same while altering features around it allows the client to practice the same oral-motor pattern over again. Second, this practice allows the client to experience success on a tremendous number of words and phrases within a short period of time. Third, it provides a wealth of practice for therapy sessions and for homework. Fourth, it encourages parents to see their child gain new skills rapidly. Finally, the speech and language pathologist in charge of this program feels good about the work because she can document that the client is gaining specific new skills each week.

When I was a junior at the University of Illinois, Professor Robert K. Simpson taught us that clients should work at a 75/25 ratio in articulation therapy: 75 percent of the work should be easy, and only 25 percent of the work should be challenging. I like this ratio, but I prefer to work at about 99/1 in R therapy. These clients need to practice a lot of perfect utterances! I love a session in which my clients practice scores of R sounds, words, phrases and sentences perfectly. I find that variety does not help, but consistency does. When making 100 productions, this could mean practicing the same word 100 times. Or it might mean rehearsing two different words fifty times each. Variety comes over time. What really matters early in treatment is persistent rehearsal of a well-controlled oral-movement pattern and a perfectly spoken cornerstone sound. The more the client says his cornerstone sound right, the greater are his chances of conquering this phoneme.

Once a basic Consonantal or Vocalic R sound is learned, most speech and language pathologists drag out the list of R words and rehearse them endlessly. But what good does it do to practice difficult words wrong? How beneficial is a session in which the client is challenged to say dozens of random words when he can say only a few of them correctly? Speech is movement, and learning the movements for R is like learning the movements of any sport. Take golf, for instance. Any golfer knows that until the swing is right, the game will be off. Thus, a golfer goes to a driving range to practice the swing, and the advice of a pro is sought to improve this skill. The determined golfer practices the swing thousands of times in order to make its movements stronger, smoother, more consistent and automatic. Speech therapy for R should be like that. It should be like being at a speech driving range. We ask our clients to rehearse the same well-produced cornerstone sound or word repeatedly in order to master it. This makes it possible for him to habituate the new oral movement and eventually to connect it to others.

~ *Summary* ~

- The difficult R client usually needs to be led step by step from his initial cornerstone sound to conversational speech.

- Clients often get stuck when we assume they are ready to produce a variety of words with R right after they have learned to say their cornerstone R.

- The key to building a successful R program for difficult clients is to identify the cornerstone sound, accept it as the first step, use it as the base of operation, and move cautiously from there. Successful R therapy for difficult clients can be accomplished by facilitating only slight variations on the cornerstone R with each subsequent step in treatment.

- The cornerstone R springs forth when all factors are right. Just because the client said the cornerstone sound once does not ensure that he will say it again any time soon. The most important thing to do with the cornerstone sound is to get the client to say it again.

- Consistent practice with the cornerstone sound creates a clear consistent production for developing more advanced skills. Failure in therapy is almost assured for tough clients when we move too quickly away from it.

- Just because a client can say his first good R sound does not mean he can hear it. Engage in activities to bring the client's own sound to his conscious auditory awareness.

- Give clear feedback about your client's productions of his cornerstone sound so he can separate correct from incorrect ones. Eliminate the gray area. Wishy-washy feedback confuses clients and prolongs therapy.

- The cornerstone word is a single word that perfectly reflects the oral-motor pattern of the cornerstone R sound. The cornerstone word is initiated once the cornerstone sound becomes consistent. Samples of cornerstone words include *are, ear, rah* or *row*.

- Teach clients to use their cornerstone word in gradually more difficult speech-motor tasks by sequencing other words around it. For example, advance from "rah" to "The fans yelled *rah*!" or, "He said *rah* when the team made the goal."

- Use the cornerstone word in rote verbal sequences to move skills toward conversation. For example, practice reciting the alphabet with correct pronunciation of letter R.

- Play verbal games that incorporate the cornerstone word so that the client learns to embed his one oral-motor pattern into other tightly controlled phonetic environments.

- Add phonemes to the cornerstone word to develop new words through mastery over the cornerstone sound. For example, advance from *are* to *art* or from *rah* to *rock*.

- Add morphemes to words in order to advance mastery skills. For example, advance from *par* to *park* to *parking* to *parking lot*.

- Test generalization skills periodically to determine if the client has begun to assimilate new patterns on his own. Add these to your practice routines.

- Clients should drill on correct R sounds in simple phonetic environments. They should avoid rehearsing a wide variety of difficult words with incorrect R sounds.

- Clients should engage in R therapy repetitively as if they were at a speech "driving range."

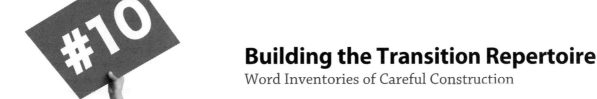

#10 Building the Transition Repertoire
Word Inventories of Careful Construction

In this chapter, our tactics of treatment are going to advance in a way that will carry our client through completion of the program. Once the oral movements of a cornerstone R sound have become sure and steady, a client is ready to move beyond. In this next phase, the client will learn to on-glide and off-glide with R in numerous ways. This is done so that he can learn to attach R's target position to the on-glide and off-glide movements of other sounds. We have referred to this as *transitioning*. The oral movement to assure successful transitions is the next level of oral-motor control the difficult R client needs.

As one speak words, phrases and sentences, one off-glides from one phoneme and on-glides into the next. The on-glide and off-glide movements of individual phonemes blend together to make new movements during these transitions. This occurs to adjacent phonemes as well as to those nearby in the sequence. Such is the *coarticulatory effect* of speech sounds. Some have used the term *sequencing* to describe this process, but I feel that that is inadequate. Sequencing phonemes conjures up the image of placing individual phonemes in a row, like one would place individual blocks in a line. Phonemes do not maintain their individual identity when lined up in words and phrases. In fact, phonemes are *unable* to maintain their separate identities when they are placed side by side in speech. Instead, each individual phoneme's movements and target position influence the other phonemes around it. New movements are created as one off-glides from one position and on-glides into another.

In the last chapter we learned to attach other sounds, syllables and words to the cornerstone sound with its single on-glide and off-glide movement pattern. Through that process, the on-glide and off-glide movements of the cornerstone sound remained the same. That is an effective way of rehearsing R early in treatment, especially for difficult clients. But the cornerstone sound can take a client only so far in R therapy. Only a small number of words contain that specific movement pattern. Ultimately, our clients must learn to on-glide and off-glide around the apex R position no matter what phonemes surround it.

DAVID

David exemplifies nicely the important task of identifying on-glide and off-glide oral-movement patterns in remediating R distortion. At the age of eleven, he came to me after two years of speech therapy for R. He had no other speech, motor or learning problems. David's therapist reported that he could produce a decent R on occasion, but that he was not getting it. She was ready to give up on him. What was wrong?

Upon examination, I found that David had been trained to produce a Tip R. He could get his tongue into position for the Tip R, and he could make an acoustically correct yet weak Vocalic R sound at the end of words. In the word-initial position, David produced a distorted Consonantal R. Deeper analysis of this distortion revealed that the problem occurred during the off-glide. After producing a good apex R sound, David made a flop forward with the tongue tip so a distorted L sound occurred on the off-glide. Whenever he tried a word that began with R, the distorted L sound interjected between the apex of R and the subsequent vowel. This additional sound on the off-glide caused R to sound distorted and it lowered overall intelligibility in rapid conversational speech. David's therapist was having him practice words with both Consonantal and Vocalic R sounds, as well as R in blends. After more than two years practicing R sounds in these uncontrolled phonetic environments, David seemed to be failing because he could not achieve a good sound on all words.

David was not failing. He had succeeded to a certain point. Specific factors were preventing him from getting any further along in the program. David was making correct on-glide movements, and he was attaining correct target position for R. Thus, he had achieved the correct acoustic quality of the R phoneme at its apex. It sounded good at the end of words. He couldn't get the initial position because his off-glide transition movements were wrong. Once I helped David understand the idea of on-gliding, hitting target position, and off-gliding without making any other sound as he transitioned into the subsequent vowel, he began to hear the added sound and was able to eliminate it. David flew through the rest of the program and was completely finished in two months.

Purpose of Chapter Ten

This is where we begin to take oral-motor therapy to an even more advanced level. David's story illustrates how viewing the production of R as a coordinated sequence of three parts is extremely important in designing appropriate treatment programs for difficult clients. In the prior three chapters, we learned techniques to get the tongue into the apex of movement for the Tip R and the Back R, and we learned to establish a cornerstone R sound. We also discussed ways to expand the client's use of his cornerstone sound by tagging other parts of speech on to it. The cornerstone sound never changed during that process even though we moved the client all the way into structured conversational speech. Now we are discussing how to help the client break up the cornerstone sound into its component parts so that all other sounds can be attached to the apex R position. The following exercises will bring clarity on this.

EXERCISE 10.1
Transition Movements of Vocalic Productions

Read aloud the following words that contain Vocalic R. Speak them very slowly by prolonging the transitionary movements of each word. Think about how your mouth is positioned for the initial sounds, and then concentrate on the flow of movement as it unfolds in transitioning to R. Say these words at a painstakingly slow pace so every detail of oral movement can be experienced. Either the Tip R or the Back R can be used for this exercise. Try both.

EAR	OR
ARE	AIR
HOUR	BURR
FEWER	TALLER
PLAYER	HAMMER
TANNER	SINGER

Did you notice how your on-glide movements toward R were somewhat different depending upon the initiating movements of the preceding sounds? An important thing happens as we speak the Vocalic R. The mouth is positioned and tensed differently for each preceding sound. Therefore, jaw, lip and tongue position begin in different ways as we glide toward the apex R position. The movement into R is slightly different with each word because the starting points are different. This difference means virtually nothing to the normal speaker and to the easy client. But these slight variations in on-glide movements reap havoc in the speech movements of the difficult R client. They are unable to adjust transitions toward and away from the apex R position.

The attempt to plan and execute a smooth sequence of two sounds that require adjustments to the transition movements between them is too much for hard clients. Either they cannot hear it or they cannot figure out how to move to make the sound correct. Their oral-movement problems make many of these clients seem apraxic as we work on R. Their planning of speech movements at this highly refined level is impaired. I have no problem classifying these clients as mildly dyspraxic because of this problem in planning and executing oral movement for R. However, standard practice in the field of speech and language pathology has never encouraged such a designation.

Further problems in R transitions ensue when a client's vowels are poorly differentiated in the first place. The intricacy of transition movements into R necessitates that our client's vowel sounds be clear and distinct no matter their phonetic environment. A client who poorly differentiates or who distorts his vowels will have no consistent places from which to on-glide into R for its vocalic productions. It will be difficult for him to learn the Vocalic R as a result.

EXERCISE 10.2
Transition Movements of Consonantal Productions

Now repeat the above exercise with consonantal productions of R. Read aloud the following words. Again, speak each word slowly while focusing on the transition movements that occur between R and the vowels. Make yourself feel each and every tiny aspect of the transitions that occur.

RAH	RIDE
READ	RAID
ROOM	RED
ROPE	RACK

Did you notice that the position for R and its off-glide was slightly different for each word? For example, did you notice the R in *room* was made with considerable lip rounding in preparation for the vowel to follow?

In the case of the Consonantal R, the client's off-glide from the initial R is influenced by the on-glide movements and apex position for the vowels that follow it. In other words, the off-glide of a Consonantal R will be produced with aspects of the subsequent vowel's on-glide movement and its apex position. Again, these glide differences are so slight that they may be imperceptible to the average reader doing the exercise the first time through. These differences will be mildly important to the easy client. As stated amply above, these movement alterations can devastate the difficult client's production of R. Oral-motor and auditory perception problems render these clients unable to position for an initial R at the same time they are preparing for the vowel or other sounds that follow. The position that will be required for the subsequent sound or series of sounds clouds his judgment about how to position for the initial R. His R position becomes compromised, and R becomes distorted. The vowels usually become distorted as well. Sometimes their ability to prepare for these shifts is so poor that the client is stymied and cannot speak.

EXERCISE 10.3
Transition Movements of Consonant Clusters

Read aloud the following words that contain basic consonant clusters. Speak them naturally, and notice your oral positions for R in each. Our samples will be for initial R blends with stops only.

Pr—praise, pretty, prune, proud
Br—brown, brain, break, bruise
Tr—train, truck, trite, trowel
Dr—drum, dream, drove, drain
Kr—cream, cram, craze, crypt
Gr—green, grass, grow, gravy

Did you notice that your oral positions for R were slightly different depending upon the initial consonant? When saying words with initial Br, the tongue is in its position for R at the same time that the lips are approximating for B. This means that the R in a Br blend contains lip closure during the on-glide phase. Let that idea sink in: We use lip closure while on-gliding into R in the Br blend! That idea is not brought up in most discussions about R therapy. In fact, every consonant that occurs before or after R influences oral position for the on-glide and off-glide movements as well as the apex position for R itself. These movement and position differences can be drastic, as in the case of Br, or they can be slight.

The Complexity of Transition Work
By now the reader may realize that there are dozens of oral-motor transitions to learn in order to speak R correctly in all contexts of words in connected speech. Complicating this work is the fact that the co-articulatory effects of one phoneme on another do not simply occur with adjacent phonemes: They occur across strings of sequential phonemes. Easy clients do not have to study and learn each and every transition that occurs in the English language. But the difficult client often has to learn a great number of these transitions individually. Naturally, such complexity requires the work to be simplified.

On-glide and off-glide transition practice can be made simple and most effective by organizing it around the vowels. Vowels are chosen for three reasons. First, transitions occur most often with vowels. Second, intelligibility rests primarily upon the vowels. Third, R is most affected by the vowels. Our work on vowel transitions will dominate treatment throughout this chapter. Consonant blends will be discussed at the end. When conquered, transition work between R and the vowels will transform a tough client into an easy one. He will develop from one who can produce only one R sound correctly, to one who can produce a correct R in virtually all phonetic environments. Transition work is essential to his success. It is his ticket out of longterm therapy.

Keep in mind that most clients cannot learn the apex of R movement alone for their cornerstone sound. Instead, most of them learn a consonantal or vocalic production of R first. They have learned to say R before or after one specific vowel. Treatment to break up the cornerstone sound always begins there.

Working with Vowel Transitions

We will begin our discussion with an "ideal" model appropriate to the phonetic understanding of speech and language pathologists. Then we will reduce this model down to one appropriate for clients. There are eleven basic vowels that are transcribed for Standard North American English: /i/, /ɪ/, /e/, /ɛ/, /æ/, /u/, /ʊ/, /o/, /ɔ/, /ɑ/ and /ʌ/ or /ə/. Beginning with the cornerstone sound, our work is to teach our clients to transition back and forth between these basic vowels and R. Keep in mind figure 10.1 when thinking through this process. All the basic English vowels are listed in the left-hand and right-hand columns, and R is presented in-between. Our clients need to learn to produce R after each vowel on the left and before each vowel on the right.

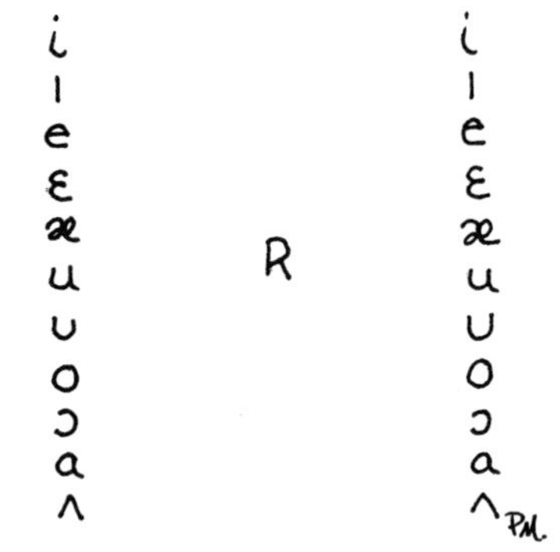

Fig. 10.1. This ideal model is useful for thinking through this process of teaching transitions, but it is far too complex for clients who do not understand phonetic transcription.

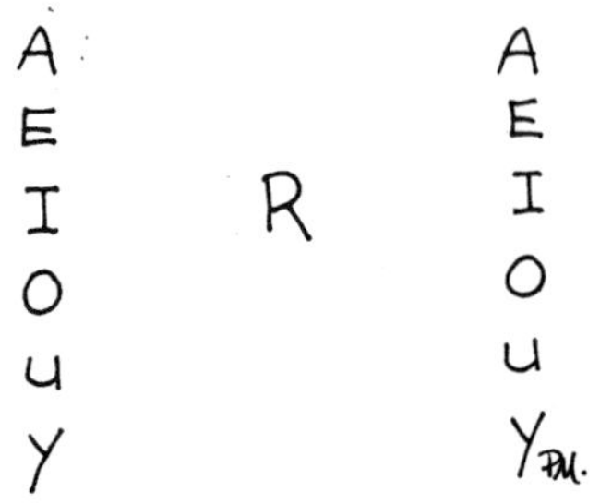

Fig. 10.2. In therapy, we must use a simplified model based on the average person's idea of vowels. Most people are taught that the vowels consist of A, E, I, O, U and sometimes Y. These six well-known vowels are listed in the left- and right-hand columns, and R appears in the middle.

These six basic letters will be the foundation of all the vowel transition work the client needs. We begin with the client's cornerstone R. The following steps are recommended:

1. Draw the simplified vowel model with the client. For example, ask, "Do you know the vowels? Can you name them?" As the client names the vowels, write them in a column from top to bottom on the left side of a page. Then write them again in a column on the right side of the page. Draw an R in-between as shown. Use bold letters so your diagram fills most of the page.

2. Select one vowel to represent the sound closest to the client's cornerstone sound. We will continue to use our example of a cornerstone sound that similar to the R in the word *are*. Demonstrate to the client how his cornerstone sound could be represented on the chart. Say, for example, "Let's use A to mean *ah*. What you can say now is 'Ah-R.'" Draw a circle around the A on the left, and another circle around the R. Connect the two with a line. Say *are* slowly as you draw your line. Repeat several times so that the client can see that the A represents the first part of his cornerstone sound and the R represents the second part. Prolong these productions so the client can hear the two parts of the cornerstone sound clearly. Make each phoneme in the cornerstone sound distinct.

Fig. 10.3.

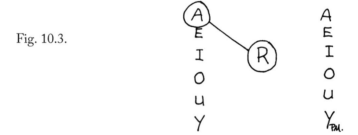

3. Ask the client to say the cornerstone sound himself as he draws a line from A to R. This will help the client understand the Ah part and the R part. You want him to see them as two separate units although he is producing it as one sound. Repeat this process several times using different colored markers for each turn so that a beautiful rainbow figure of colored lines is drawn. With each turn, give immediate feedback using clear terms for correct and incorrect productions. Don't let your client get away with poor productions here. He can say his cornerstone sound well, so make him do it. This work is a repetition of the cornerstone work taught earlier. As such, this step can be used early in therapy when the cornerstone sound is first learned.

Fig. 10.4.

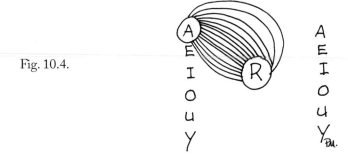

4. Teach the client to make transitions from his cornerstone sound to other vowels on the other side of R. Begin this process by circling the same vowel on the other side of the chart. Following our example, we circle A in the right-hand column. Now ask the client to say his cornerstone sound and the identical vowel on the other side of R in a three-part sequence. This would be "Ah-R-Ah." By this time, the client's cornerstone sound should be consistent and true. He should be able to say this neatly. However, the presence of the new sound on the other side of the cornerstone sound my trip him up. He may mispronounce the cornerstone sound. Slow him down to make sure the cornerstone sound stays true.

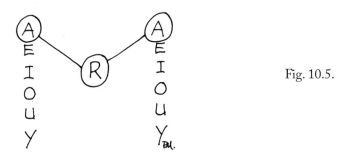

Fig. 10.5.

5. Some clients will be able to maintain voice while transitioning from their cornerstone sound to a vowel on the other side of the sequence. But many will not. Allow your client to break voice wherever he needs to in order to regroup for the next sound in the sequence. Require only that the client make the cornerstone sound and the one additional sound. Rehearse this sequence several times if he is producing it well. If not, try another combination.
6. Try another combination by moving on to another vowel to use in sequence with the cornerstone sound. Following our example, one might select O. Ask the client to say "Ah-R-O." Give ample time for the client to sequence slowly and as best he can.

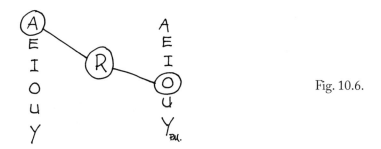

Fig. 10.6.

7. Test each vowel in this way to find the ones that can be pronounced well. Over time, the client will learn to make all these transitions. Build them slowly and carefully. Rehearse the ones he can do well, and ignore the others. Allow him to break voice and regroup at any point in the sequences. Remember to work at a high rate of success. Consistent practice of perfect sound combinations is your goal.

The Revelations of Vowel Transition Work
The transition work reveals several subtle things about a hard client's pronunciation skills. Any vowels that are slightly distorted become glaringly obvious. These vowels must be fixed. Never let a client get away with vowel distortion in this transition work. More damage will be done and stagnation will occur if the vowels remain muddy. Stop working on R for a while, and rehearse in isolation the vowels that are in error. You will have to do substantial auditory discrimination work here so the client can hear the vowels as distinct sounds and recognize slight distortions. Then begin to incorporate the R work back in as each vowel stabilizes with a good sound. If necessary, spend part of many sessions rehearsing the vowels alone. Do not work on these vowels in syllables or words. Work in isolation only, and prolong them so that the client can begin to hear them well.

The so-called *short vowels* are not appropriate for this transition, because they cannot be prolonged. The easiest way to do this work is with vowels that develop early and prolong easily. These are the *long vowels*. Thus, the following vowel sounds are used:

- For A, use the Ah as in *Bah*
- For E, use the E as in *Bee*
- For I, use I as in *Bye*
- For O, use O as in *Boat*
- For U, use Oo as in *Boot*

We must pay careful attention to jaw movements during this vowel transition work. Often, jaw instability is the cause of sound distortion. Include activities to increase awareness and control of the jaw and to stabilize it at midline, if necessary. Do not hold the jaw to restrict its movements. That is a passive and relatively ineffective way to facilitate jaw stability. The client will relax the jaw muscles to allow you to have control over it. Instead, give the client something thin on which to bite during this speech practice. Have him bite with the molars on the handle of a Toothette®. This will stabilize the jaw in a partially graded open position. Biting down on a thin object is a much better technique to facilitate jaw stability. It encourages the client to keep the jaw elevated as its muscles activate.

Even if the vowels are well-spoken in isolation, distortion may occur during the transition exercises. This is a reflection of what happens to his transitions when R occurs in connected speech. To learn how to maintain clarity on the vowels while transitioning with R is the work that straightens all this out. Intelligibility improves as the vowels begin to retain their distinct acoustic properties in connected speech. In fact, parents often report that their child sounds much better after these rehearsals, even when R is still in its early stages. Work slowly and carefully, and have the client clearly articulate all the sounds so that they are distinct.

If you notice your client cannot make certain transitions at all, he may need more time working on the cornerstone sound. Incorporate vowel drill alongside this work so that the client can begin to tune the ear better. Have the client produce the sounds in sequence without voicing in-between. Also, consider doing this work with the other glides—L, Y and W—and not just R in order to make more comparisons and contrasts. This will help you build toward these transitions.

Be mindful that certain transitions require the insertion of Y or W. For example, in producing R after long E (as in the word *ear*), a Y sound is inserted. We do not say "E-R," we say "E-Y-R." These sequences need to be practiced as more complicated sequences.

Our goal in this area is to help our clients learn to produce all vowel sequences with R. Make notes about which ones he can and cannot do. Rehearse the ones he can do, and teach him the others. Each session of therapy should include some work on these transitions. Begin with the transitions you are sure he can do well. Gradually move into the sequences that are more challenging. Draw new charts as needed. The goal of this work is for the client to learn to make each and every transition. Some transitions will be learned immediately. Others may take months to conquer.

Voicing and Silence During Transition Practice
The beginning transition work must be analyzed and adjusted to each client. It ultimately must be done by maintaining voice while moving from one sound to the other, the most advanced way to practice. However, for difficult R clients a problem occurs in the transition. The client distorts the transition by adding other sounds to it as he moves clumsily from his cornerstone sound to other vowels or consonants. This gets down to the core of his oral-motor problem. The client does not know how to move correctly from R to other sounds or from other sounds to R in a straight line. As a result, other vowel and consonant sounds are heard in the midst of the transitions, which cause the listener to hear R as a distortion even if the apex position of R has been attained.

This problem was illustrated in the story of David that appeared in the opening section of this chapter. Transition distortions come in all forms. Most of these added sounds are simple distortion of R and the true vowels or they are additions of the other glides—W, L and Y. Periodic transition problems include consonant distortions as widely divergent as the addition of V or Z.

To solve this problem, the transition is performed in silence. We do this by voicing on the cornerstone R and the vowel to be attached to it, and by remaining silent or voiceless during the transition. A moment of silence during the transition movement eliminates the distorted element. What is left is the production of a clear vowel and a clear R. We want our clients to hear the clear vowel and the clear R apex in isolation in a simple sequence. This allows him to hear what the Vocalic or Consonantal R should sound like when it occurs in a sequence with the incorrect transition element absent. Gradually, we ask the client to keep voicing throughout the transitions and we train his ear to hear the unnecessary sound that occurs. Once he can hear this unwanted sound, he can work to eliminate it.

Transition problems are the main reason clients remain stuck in longterm R therapy. These clients are allowed to rehearse a great number of words with uncontrolled phonetic environments. As a result, they are adding unnecessary sound to their transitions.

This problem is apparent right in the initial call made by referring therapists or parents. The caller will report that the client can do it but that he "still has trouble with some words." What they mean is that the client can produce a good apex R sound but he cannot make all the necessary transitions. The client needs a systematic approach to learning how to transition with R and every basic vowel. He needs to do this work at the syllable and the simple word level. He also needs to work in silence and in voice until the transitions are conquered.

Words with Transitions to Vocalic R

Vowel transition work advances from nonsense word repetition to meaningful words. These words should completely reflect the transition work the client is accomplishing with the vowel charts, and they should reflect the client's vocabulary level. For example, if the client can sequence Ah-R, he is ready to practice saying the words *are, bar, jar* and *star*. Rehearsal of these words should be done at a slow rate so that the client has enough time to make the transition between vowel and R with perfect articulation and no additional sounds. The client should be encouraged to say each simple word as if it had two syllables: the vowel and the R. He should be allowed to break his voice in the transition if necessary.

The following words are good selections for working on the Vocalic R with the five basic vowels—A, E, I, O, U. The reader will recognize that some of these words, when *super-articulated* in this way, actually do not represent how the average person pronounces them. We are doing this extremely precise work to help the client straighten out his auditory perception and to control his oral movements for the individual sounds. Later, he can slur them a little like everyone else. These are basic words that reflect specific oral-motor patterns.

WORDS TO PRACTICE WHEN AH-R EMERGES	PRONUNCIATION
are	Ah-R
bar	Bah-R
car	Cah-R
far	Fah-R
jar	Jah-R

mar	Mah-R
par	Pah-R
star	Stah-R
tar	Tah-R
tsar	Zah-R

WORDS TO PRACTICE WHEN E-R EMERGES	PRONUNCIATION
ear	Ee-R
deer	Dee-R
hear	Hee-R
here	Hee-R
pier	Pee-R
steer	Stee-R
we're	Wee-R

WORDS TO PRACTICE WHEN I-R EMERGES	PRONUNCIATION
fire	Fi-R
flier	Fli-R
higher	Hi-R
liar	Li-R
mire	Mi-R
pyre	Pi-R
sire	Si-R
tire	Ti-R
wire	Wi-R

WORDS TO PRACTICE WHEN O-R EMERGES	PRONUNCIATION
or	Oh-R
bore	Boh-R
core	Coh-R
door	Doh-R
for	Foh-R
four	Foh-R
more	Moh-R
poor	Poh-R
store	Stoh-R
wore	Woh-R

WORDS TO PRACTICE WHEN U-R EMERGES	PRONUNCIATION
cure	Cu-R
pure	Pu-R
sure	Shu-R

tour	Tou-R
you're	You-R

Words with Transitions from Consonantal R

Select more words to rehearse as each consonantal transition skill emerges. For example, as the client demonstrates ability to transition from R to Oh, practice saying the words *robe, wrote* and *rose*. These words should be simple in terms of phonetic content, and they should reflect the client's vocabulary level. Rehearsal should be done at a very slow rate so that the client gives himself enough time to make the transition with perfect sound and nothing added. These words should be pronounced as if they had three syllables, with R as its own syllable. These can be made with a smooth voiced transition or with voice broken in the transition.

The following words are good selections for working on the Consonantal R with the five basic vowels:

WORDS TO PRACTICE WHEN R-AH EMERGES	PRONUNCIATION
Rob	R-Ah-B
rock	R-Ah-K
rod	R-Ah-D
Ron	R-Ah-N
rot	R-Ah-T

WORDS TO PRACTICE WHEN R-E EMERGES	PRONUNCIATION
reach	R-E-Ch
read	R-E-D
reef	R-E-F
reek	R-E-K
ream	R-E-M
reap	R-E-P

WORDS TO PRACTICE WHEN R-I EMERGES	PRONUNCIATION
ride	R-I-D
rife	R-I-F
rhyme	R-I-M
ripe	R-I-P
right	R-I-T

WORDS TO PRACTICE WHEN R-O EMERGES	PRONUNCIATION
robe	R-Oh-B
road	R-Oh-D
rogue	R-Oh-G
roam	R-Oh-M
rope	R-Oh-P

rose	R-Oh-Z
wrote	R-Oh-T

WORDS TO PRACTICE WHEN R-U EMERGES	PRONUNCIATION
rube	R-Oo-B
rude	R-Oo-D
roof	R-Oo-F
room	R-Oo-M
root	R-Oo-T
Ruth	R-Oo-Th

Introduce Morphemes to the Root Words

Add morphemes to the basic words practiced above in order to make them more difficult. For example, expand from the root word *room* to *rooms, roomy, rooming* and *roomer*. The client will continue to rehearse the basic oral-motor pattern with small, new movements added to the end of it. Morphemes that can be added include:

MORPHEME	EXAMPLE
Plural—s	road, roads
Possessive—s	Ron, Ron's
Third Person Verb	reap, reaps
Present Progressive Verb	root, rooting
Past Tense	root, rooted
Adjective—ly	right, rightly
Adjective—y or ie	rose, rosie
Comparative—er	roomy, roomier
Superlative—est	ripe, ripest
Diminutive—y or ie	Rob, Robbie
Diminutive- ette	rose, rosette

Then, place these basic words with their morphemes into simple sentences. For example, place *room, roomy, roomier* and *roomiest* into three sentences: "My room is roomy. This room is roomier. That room is the roomiest." Construct sentences void of other R words in order to focus on the target sounds and words at hand.

Conjugate R Verbs

Like adding morphemes to root words, R words that are verbs can be conjugated as a way to practice the same oral-motor pattern many times in a row.

TO RIDE

am riding	am not riding	
are riding	are not riding	aren't riding
do ride	do not ride	don't ride

did ride	did not ride	didn't ride
can ride	cannot ride	can't ride
will ride	will not ride	won't ride
could ride	could not ride	couldn't ride
would ride	would not ride	wouldn't ride
should ride	should not ride	shouldn't ride
might ride	might not ride	mightn't ride
could have ridden	could not have ridden	couldn't have ridden
should have ridden	should not have ridden	shouldn't have ridden
would have ridden	would not have ridden	wouldn't have ridden
might have ridden	might not have ridden	mightn't have ridden

I hope the reader can see the tremendous number of phrases that can be practiced. This type of work gives us powerful lists to train specific oral-motor patterns repeatedly within a short period of time. Once practiced alone, these conjugated verb phrases can be placed into simple sentences. For example, place the verb phrase *cannot ride* into:

- The boy cannot ride his bike.
- The man cannot ride in his car.
- The woman cannot ride too soon.
- The jockey cannot ride his steed.
- The dog cannot ride in the wagon.

Make these sentences void of any other words that contain R. Practice them in a lilting pattern, with similar intonation and stress patterns on each one. When ready, your client should be able to practice them with a high degree of success. This work will help stabilize his oral-motor patterns. Ultimately, these kinds of exercises will bring speed and accuracy together for conversational speech.

Multisyllabic Words and Phrases with Vocalic Transitions
Build slightly more difficult work by expanding into multisyllabic words. For example, expand from *bar* to *barbell, barley* and *barbeque*. Remember, the simple words are not root words, *per se*, so the expanded words will have no conceptual connection to the base words. Instead, the base words represent basic oral-motor patterns, and the expanded words represent increased movement demands on those patterns. In this way, the client will continue to rehearse the same oral-motor transition pattern he has already learned, but he will be working from a much bigger vocabulary set and the transition work will be somewhat more demanding.

Continue to work slowly, and allow the client to break the words up into distinct syllables. Encourage him to separate R into its own syllable. There are hundreds of words that fit these patterns, especially if you expand to phrases of five syllables or more. These will give you a start:

BASIC PATTERN	TWO-SYLLABLE WORDS	THREE+SYLLABLE WORDS AND PHRASES
are	argue, arcade, archer arbor, army, artist	artichoke, arsenic, artifact article, artisan, artistry
bar	barbell, barber, barcode barfly, barter, barley	barbarous, barbecue, barrio barberry, barbershop, bartender
car	cartoon, carton, carbon carcass, car coat, cargo	carnival, carbonate, carnivore carbuncle, cardinal
far	Far East, far out, farm house, farm yard	far away, far-reaching, farsighted
mar	market, marble, marshal martial, Martian, marvel	martingale, martial law, marsupial marzipan, marvelous
par	party, parcel, pardon parfait, parka, parking	parcel post, parliament, parmesan parsonage, participate, particle
tar	tardy, target, Tarmac tarnish, tarpon	tartar sauce, tardier, targeted tarnishing

Rehearse these words alone and in simple sentences void of other R words, such as:

- Mark went to the market and marveled at the Martian.
- Pardon me. I must park at the party.
- The farmhouse was far out in the farm yard.
- Don't argue with artichokes! They have an army!

Multisyllabic Words and Phrases with Consonantal Transitions

This activity includes a change from the vocalic to the consonantal base pattern. As each consonantal transition is acquired, build slightly more difficult work by expanding into multisyllabic words and phrases that incorporate the same base oral-motor pattern. For example, expand from *reef* to *refine* and *refer*. Again, these are not root words and the expanded words will have no meaningful connection to the base word. These are oral-motor patterns of increasing complexity.

Continue to work rather slowly. Allow the client to break the words up into distinct syllables, if necessary. Encourage him to separate R into its own syllable. There also are hundreds of words that fit these patterns, and more so if you move toward phrases of five or more syllables. The following two-, three- and four-syllable words and phrases will give you a start. Please note that many of these words contain a change in syllable divisions and accent. Still, the same essential oral-motor pattern is required within each set. Also, some of these words contain other R sounds that need to be ignored.

BASIC PATTERN	EXPANSIONS ON THE BASE PATTERN
rob	Robbie, robbing, robin, Robin Hood
rock	rocky, Rock-n-roll, rock bottom, rocket, rock salt
rot	rotten, rotting, Rottterdam
reach	recharge, rechart, recheck, rechargable

read	redo, redeem, redress, redemption, redistrict, reduce, reduction,
reef	refer, reflect, refine, referral, refinement, reflector, refill, reflex, reflexive, reforest, refreshment
reek	reeky, reclaim, record, rekindle, reclaiming, recombine, recap, recall, recant, recorder, recount, recover
ream	remain, remand, remark, remainder, remember, remission, remind, remiss, remote, remittance, remodel, removing
reap	repeat, repass, repay, repacking, repeating, repack, repaint, repair, reposing
ride	riding, rider, ridership, Ridell
rhyme	rhyming, rhymer, rhyming word
ripe	ripen, ripest, ripening
right	right hand, righteous, right handed, right of way, rightful, rightly, right wing, right winger
robe	robot, robust, Robocop, robotman
road	rodeo, roadway, road sign, Rodeo, rodent, Rodin
roam	romance, Roman, romaine, romantic, Roman Number, Romeo
rope	roping, rope rider, Rope-a-Dope
rose	rosebud, rosebush, rosette, rosary, rosemary, rose water
rote	rotate, rotund, rotunda, wrote
rube	Rubens, rubric, ruby, rubella, rubicund, Rubic Cube
rude	rudely, rudeness, rudiment
roof	rooftop, roofing, roofer, roof garden
rule	ruling, ruler, ruling class, rule of thumb
room	roomer, rooming, roomful, room and board, roommate
root	rootbeer, rootstock

Rehearse these words alone and then in simple sentences void of other R words if possible. For example, rehearse:

- The record was recovered.
- The ripest tomato is ripening.
- Coach always says, "Repeat, replay and repair!"
- Romeo was a romantic who loved romance.

Create New Phrases and Sentences with the New Sequences
Now the client should be able to stretch his skill further by rehearsing these motor patterns as they occur across words. Use your imagination for these. For example, if Rah is his cornerstone sound, and the client has begun to rehearse sequences like A-Rah, E-Rah, I-Rah, O-Rah and U-Rah, these might be expanded into the following:

- A-Rah: I ate a rotten peach.
- E-Rah: He robbed the man.
- I-Rah: I rocked the audience.

- O-Rah: G<u>o ro</u>ck the baby.
- U-Rah: I'm talking to <u>you, R</u>on.

A simple list of five sentences like this makes for good homework. It should take the client less than one minute to read these sentences aloud with good cornerstone R sounds. He can say them twice per day between weekly therapy sessions for a total of 60 practices (5 sentences x 2 practices per day x 6 days). The list can be memorized easily for more practice throughout the day. Imagine if your client repeated these five sentences six times every day before his next appointment. He would have practiced the basic vowel sequences 180 times before you saw him again. That is a lot of practice! These are outstanding homework activities that will ensure rapid success. Make sure there are no other R words in the sentences.

Build Fluidity and Rhythm of Movement
Once the client has begun to sequence around R with several different vowels, he is ready to learn to move fluidly and rhythmically through repetitions of his basic transitions. For example, once he can say "Ah-R-Ah," he must learn to transition multiple times in sequence by practicing "Ah-R-Ah-R-Ah-R-Ah-R." The difference between the single sequence and the repeated sequence is like the difference between taking one step and walking. Taking one step is good, but you will never get anywhere unless you can walk. Positioning for a step is a static movement, but walking is a dynamic movement process. Walking through a sequence of same transitions is what builds fluidity and rhythm of movement. This is how the client bonds the movements of R into a stream of connected movements. This helps the transitions sound more natural. It can be very important work for successful carryover of correct R productions into spontaneous conversational speech.

Sequential transitioning work is a process of learning to *babble* with R. Babbling is the rhythmic production of sequences of consonants and vowels usually seen in babies. One usually thinks of it as early developing consonants, like B, M, D or W. But babbling also includes primitive forms of later developing sounds, like L and R. Vocal babies babble intensively between six and eighteen months of age. They can be heard babbling with a huge variety of consonants and vowels. Babbling is a baby's way of having fun with long speech sequences before many of his real words emerge. Transition work at this level of R therapy is a sophisticated process of babbling with R. I like to call it *systematic babbling*. We select only those transitions that are produced perfectly for work on these fluid sequences. We begin work slowly so that the client can say each component of the longer strings perfectly. We do not compromise accuracy of production for speed of sequence.

One of the great problems in clients with longterm persistent R misarticulation is an inability to produce connected speech with good rate and rhythm. Another is the habitual use of a fast rate of speech—too fast to support the client's oral-motor ability. In normal development, babbling begins *arhythmically*, meaning "without rhythm." The baby who is just beginning to babble produces one clumsy syllable after another in a loosely knit sequence. But babbling soon becomes bouncy, well-timed and rhythmic. Speech rhythm is the uniform beat in syllables and words. *Beat* is the periodic production of pulses or throbs in speech. We are all familiar with the beat of music. By slowing down and overfocusing on the beat and rhythm of syllable and word productions in babbling utterances with R, we help our clients learn to produce R's on-glide and off-glide movements with fluidly and rhythm just like a baby does naturally.

Better rhythm can be accomplished by producing speech models with over-exaggerated and distinct beat properties. We punch out the vowel and the initial cornerstone R as if each were its own syllable, and we help our clients do likewise. We can choose a specific intonation pattern (*ala,* Melodic Intonation Therapy) to make the syllabic nature of each utterance stand out. We can use hand and arm gestures and facial expressions to highlight these beat properties.

A focus on rhythm does not have to wait for these advanced levels of training. It can and should be added liberally any time throughout all levels of treatment, especially with those clients who demonstrate dysarthric speech patterns. The persistence of well-paced rate, exaggerated beats, flawless rhythm, punctuated syllables and regular intonation patterns on our models helps the client look beyond R and focus on the transition process. The client can hear the transitions more easily when we regularize these prosodic elements in our own model utterances. Further, clients can produce these transitions more clearly and consistently when they adopt these strategies for themselves.

Babbling sequences can be rehearsed at any time of day or night and under any circumstances. Your client can repeat them while in the shower, bath or bed; while riding in a car; or watching television. He can mouth them silently during quiet times at home or school. Consider assigning homework for your client to repeat selected babbling sequences twice per day between weekly sessions. Help him make a list of all the places where he might be able to do this.

Add Speed to Oral Movement
Add speed to transition productions once the client can make correct transitions consistently. Remember, up until now we have stressed the importance of allowing the client to work as slowly as necessary. We have stated that treatment routines should sacrifice speed for accuracy. Now, it is time to increase speed while maintaining accuracy. We continue with the same fluidity and rhythm work as described above, but we challenge the client to make these utterances just a little bit faster and more naturally. Do not speed things up too quickly. Accuracy is the key. When accuracy of sound production wanes, or when transitions become sloppy, slow down again. This is not a race. We simply are trying to bring the client's rate of speech in this work up to a normal rate. You will find that your clients will be able to speed up on some transitions but not others. That is to be expected. It will be common to say, "Say this one as fast as you can," and, "Slow down on that one so that you say it perfectly."

Despite the fact that we want to maintain accuracy most of the time, there are times to practice these sequences so fast that lots of pronunciation errors occur. Help your client see these wild utterances as humorous by showing delight in his attempt to go so fast that he makes lots of errors. "Whew! You went so fast on that one that all the correct R's went away!" This type of *negative practice* will help him see his speed limit. He will experience the drastic difference between his ability to pronounce R under conditions that are very slow and very fast. He will learn how to adjust his speed to pronounce R well under the demands of various conversational speech situations. His productions will become faster and he will maintain accuracy throughout.

It has been my consistent experience that something special occurs when clients can begin to make good transitions with consistent fluency and a rate that is approaching normal. These skills begin to transfer into the oral movements of conversational speech. Correct R begins to appear sporadically as if it were sprinkled into the discourse. The right acoustic quality of R will appear during conversation because the client will begin to move automatically with them. With speed and accuracy, a client begins to incorporate his new oral-movement patterns into his pre-existing ones. I have worked with many clients who leapt successfully into conversation using correct R sounds without ever having practiced one single R word after they conquered rate, rhythm and fluidity. The transition work teaches a client to move into and out of R within varying phonetic contexts during rapid speech movement sequences. Once a basic R sound has been learned during earlier stages of treatment, transition work becomes the focus of the oral-motor training. And once these skills are learned, clients will have acquired all they need to drop the movements of R into their conversational speech motor patterns.

Build Transitions with Consonants Carefully
Many clients will need specific work on consonant clusters containing R. These patterns usually are reflected in the client's personal set of "The Hardest Words in the World." Therefore, refer back to this list frequently as you work through this section. The clusters should be reassessed after substantial work on the vowel transitions is complete. Many of the consonant clusters will emerge spontaneously as the client gains control over the vowel transitions. Therefore, we retest the consonant clusters now to discover which ones have already made it into the client's spontaneous repertoire. Identify those that have already been acquired and those that will need specific training. The following recommendations are made for addressing the transition work of consonant clusters.

1. Begin R-cluster work with those clusters that have emerged spontaneously, in order to solidify them and make them automatic. Make sure the client can use the already changed clusters on a wide variety of words, both simple and complex. For example, if the initial Gr blend of the word *green* has emerged, make sure to work on a wide variety of other words, such as *grow, grass, aggravate, agriculture, anger* and so forth.
2. Make cluster work easier by stretching R-blends into full syllables. For example, make Dr into the syllable *der*. Rehearse *drum* as "der-um."
3. Remember that some clients will have learned their first R in a specific consonant cluster. Treat that cluster as the cornerstone sound and move forward with it as described throughout this and our previous chapter.
4. Consider teaching the R clusters in a specific sequence:

A. Train clients to produce each phoneme of the clusters in isolation.
B. Teach clients to perform clusters with voiced transition movements.
C. Teach clients to say the consonant and R simultaneously so the productions sound like mature clusters.

5. Some blends with R will be easy to learn; others will be difficult. Don't worry about these differences. Overrehearse the easy ones. Put off the hard ones until the client has gained better overall control of R.
6. Some difficult clients are able to learn only one cluster for a long time. Do not think of this as failure. It is success to a certain degree. Continue to rehearse this cluster, move on to other aspects of the program, and return to the other clusters later.
7. Some R-blends are very difficult to accomplish with a Tip R. For example, the Dr blend is quite difficult because the tip must articulate with the alveolus for the D, and then shoot back to the velar area for the R. The same is true for the tongue movements in the Tr blend. For this reason, the Tip R is viewed as an inferior way of producing R. It slows down connected speech movements. Practice these clusters by adding the schwa and stretching the cluster into a full syllable. Slow down the productions considerably. Consider switching to the Back R when you begin work on clusters, but remember that the Back R will be unobtainable by a great number of clients. Sometimes the Back R will emerge several years after the Tip R has become established in connected speech.
8. Practice R clusters with all stops:

   - Pr—press, pray
   - Br—brown, brain
   - Tr—train, truck
   - Dr—drum, drink
   - Kr—crumb, crack
   - Gr—green, grass

9. Practice R clusters with the fricatives:

   - Fr—friend, frown
   - Vr—vroom!
   - Shr—shred, Shrek
   - Thr—three, throw

10. Practice three-consonant initial clusters:

    - Spr—spring, sprout, sprain
    - Str—street, stretch, strong
    - Scr—scream, scratch, screw

11. Practice medial and final clusters. Regardless of where the actual syllable break occurs, the on-glide and off-glide transition movements between R and the other consonants must be learned. These include:

   R WITH STOPS
   - /ɚ·p/—carp, car pool
   - /ɚ·b/—herb, curbside
   - /ɚ·t/—hurt, horticulture
   - /ɚ·d/—word, orderly
   - /ɚ·k/—park, harken
   - /ɚ·g/—iceberg, organize

   R WITH NASALS
   - /ɚ·m/—harm, farmer
   - /ɚ·n/—burn, Arnold

   R WITH FRICATIVES AND AFFRICATIVES
   - /ɚ·f/—scarf, curfew
   - /ɚ·b/—nerve, nervous
   - /ɚ·s/—horse, herself
   - /ɚ·z/—cars, ours
   - /ɚ·ʃ/—harsh, harshly
   - /ɚ·ʒ/—Persian
   - /ɚ·tʃ/—church, perching
   - /ɚ·dʒ/—urge, urgent
   - /ɚ·θ/—worth, orthoptic
   - /ɚ·ð/—worthy

   THREE-CONSONANT FINAL R CLUSTERS
   - /ɚ·ps/—burps
   - /ɚ·bs/—suburbs
   - /ɚ·ts/—hurts
   - /ɚ·ds/—herds
   - /ɚ·ks/—perks
   - /ɚ·gs/—Borgs
   - /ɚ·ms/—terms
   - /ɚ·ns/—burns

12. Work on R clusters that occur across words. All of the clusters listed above can be employed in this manner. Consider the following:

   - /ɚ·b/—the sto<u>re b</u>y the gas station
   - /br/—the ca<u>b r</u>ight outside

- /ɚs/—my fou<u>r s</u>ocks
- /sr/—Mi<u>ss R</u>osswell
- /tr/—boa<u>t r</u>ide
- /ɚʃ/—ti<u>re sh</u>op
- /ɚð/—this o<u>r th</u>at

Isolate the Apex Position

The ultimate key to successful R therapy lies in a client's ability to produce R in isolation so that he can sound out any word with R. The apex of R movement must be teased away from other attached vowel or consonant movements. When the cornerstone sound is strong and automatic and the work of this chapter is underway, we can begin to teach the client to break up his cornerstone sound into two distinct parts: the R part and the transitionary vowel or consonant part. This isolates the acoustic quality of R heard at the apex of speech movement. Once isolated, this true R can be used in any position of any word. When this was previously introduced it was experimental, to give the client an added element of practice. Now we must expect the client to execute this skill in order to isolate the R apex for use in all words that contain R.

How do we isolate the R sound? Begin this training from the outset of treatment. Throughout all our work, slow down transitions so much that the client can hear the two distinct sounds of his cornerstone sound. A slow production allows the client ample time to hear the two distinct parts. Second, teach him how to isolate the apex R sound by breaking our voice between the apex and the adjacent on-glide or off-glide. Ask the client to do the same. This is the silent transition discussed above. If the client can break voice between the on-glide or off-glide and the apex position, then he will have succeeded to produce an isolated R sound. The difficult client becomes a significantly easier one once he can produce an isolated apex R sound consistently. The ability to produce the sound of R in isolation marks the beginning of taking control of R in all contexts. This skill will bring R therapy into its final phase. And, by the way, this is the skill that has made the easy client a breeze from the beginning.

Make R a Full Syllable

Once the apex of the R sound can be produced at will and the real isolated R can be uttered, the client will be ready to sound out any word. This is where we must be careful. It is easy to assume we can push forward willy-nilly into any word. Again, difficult clients will be unable to do so. That is because their transitions skills will continue to break down as soon as additional levels of complexity are added to the work. We must help these difficult clients learn to pronounce words as if R were its own syllable. For example, the one-syllable word *deer* is pronounced "dee-r," with a break where the dash appears. Likewise:

- *Car* will be pronounced "ca-er"
- *Throw* will be pronounced "th-er-ow"
- *Pardon* will be pronounced "pa-er-don"
- *Card* will be pronounced "ca-er-d"

The break allows him time to slip into and out of the R position without worrying about gliding smoothly. And it helps him keep vowels clear. With the ability to isolate the apex of R, the client is ready to pronounce any word with R. Many clients beam when they reach this stage. They know that they now have the skill to try any word. They can go back to their list of "The Hardest Words in the World" and begin to sound them out. Don't let your clients get discouraged because they have to pronounce these difficult words slowly. Assure them that they will get better and faster with time.

1. Practice counting number sequences heavily loaded with R words. For example, once the client can pronounce *thirty* as *th-er-ty*, he can count from 30 to 39 like this:

   - th-er-ty
   - th-er-ty-one
   - th-er-ty-two
   - th-er-ty-th-er-ee
   - th-er-ty-fou-er
   - th-er-ty-five
   - th-er-ty-six
   - th-er-ty-seven
   - th-er-ty-eight
   - th-er-ty-nine

2. Practice other number sequences with *thirty* or *forty*. For example, have the client count from 40–49, 130–139, 140–149, 330–339, 440–449, and so forth. Alternately, ask your clients to practice sequences like 23, 33, 43, 53, 63, 73, 83, 93, 103, and 113. Kids who love math get enthusiastic about this type of work. They busy themselves coming up with new sequences to practice. Number sequences like this allow a client to drill on the same oral-motor pattern repeatedly until he can do so fluidly. Work slowly, break R into its own syllable and build speed over time. Have fun with breakdowns that occur at fast rates so the client can learn how to slow down under his own volition.

3. Practice words that end with an *er* suffix by turning verbs into nouns. For example, change *wash* to *washer* and *throw* into *thrower*. Play a fill-in-the-blank game to generate these words. "Someone who washes clothes is a . . ." and the client answers with the appropriate noun: washer. This way the client takes control of his spontaneous productions of R while his mind searches for the new word. Practice such words alone and in simple sentences void of other R sounds. For example, the client might practice "Someone who washes clothes is a clothes washer." Here are a few samples:

player	driver	reader	eater
jumper	thrower	catcher	drinker

dancer	washer	singer	writer
bouncer	waver	teacher	painter
rider	walker	tanner	bather
planter	planner	feeder	sitter

4. Practice the titles of sports figures that end in *er*. Break *er* into its own syllable at first. Gradually make a transition between the root word and the suffix. Finally, shorten the transition time so that the word sounds more natural. Practice these alone and embedded in real sentences void of other R sounds. There are hundreds of words and phrases like this, many of which introduce R in other positions. Here are a few samples:

catcher	skate boarder	surfer
pitcher	rock climber	jogger
hitter	snow border	marathoner
race car driver	pole vaulter	walker
swimmer	boxer	hurtler
weight lifter	skier	sky diver
pitcher	runner	golfer

5. Practice more words with an *er* suffix by using comparatives. Use these alone and in simple sentences void of other R sounds. Here are a few samples:

newer	younger	prettier	funnier
cleaner	brighter	chewier	uglier
lighter	sooner	thirstier	earlier
nicer	harder	happier	hungrier
older	easier	tastier	lonelier
later	busier	dirtier	heavier

6. Practice the titles of family members by isolating the *er* at the end.

mother	grandmother	mother-in law	father
grandfather	father-in-law	sister	step-sister
sister-in-law	brother	step-brother	brother-in-law

The Special Work of R and L

Throughout most of these exercises, most of our sample words have been devoid of one specific phoneme: L. This is because the transition process between R and L is the most difficult. Many of our clients have difficulty with both because R and L can be difficult to discriminate and their oral-motor patterns can be easily confused. Young children often treat all four glides—W, L, Y, R—as if they were one single sound, readily interchanging them. In essence, the four glides are the same sound made in different places in the mouth.

W is made at the lips. L is made with the tongue tip extended to the alveolus. Y is made with the body of the tongue stretching toward the palate. And R is made with the tip or the back of the tongue stretching toward the velum. All four phonemes sound similar.

The ability to clearly differentiate all four glides is the heart of the longterm persistent R misarticulation, and many of our clients are still operating with this confusion. Words that contain both L and R often are on the client's list of the "Hardest Words in the World," often including *world, squirrel, girl, pearl, early* and the like.

Successful R therapy for most clients needs to include special work on words that contain both R and L. We do this from the outset of therapy by working on all four glides in isolation. Over time, our clients learn to differentiate all four sounds and to produce each one clearly. Toward the end of treatment they will be able to produce words and phrases that contain any and all of the glides sequenced together.

The following ideas are presented from easiest to most difficult. The easy ones should be introduced early in treatment, and the difficult ones should be presented toward the end. An individual client's ability to move through these steps can be a nice way to monitor progress in treatment.

1. Make sure that your client is producing W, L and Y correctly. And make sure that L is produced with the tongue tip stretching up to the alveolar ridge. Do not accept productions of L with interdental tongue placement. Make sure your client does not flop the tongue forward once the alveolus has been tapped for L. This is the result of a loose and floppy tongue. Include techniques to improve overall tension in the tongue. Also include techniques to facilitate jaw stability. An unstable jaw usually goes hand in hand with a loose and floppy tongue.
2. Practice single syllables with all four glides. Work the phonemes from front to back in the following sequence: W, L, Y, R. The front-to-back relationship of these sounds will become apparent to your client. Focus on the unique oral position and auditory quality for each glide.

   - wah, lah, yah, rah
   - woh, loh, yoh, roh
   - wee, lee, yee, ree
   - woo, loo, yoo, roo

3. Practice rhyming real words with W, L, Y and R. Practice them alone at first, and in phrases or sentences later. Continue to focus on the unique oral position and auditory quality for each glide. Emphasize place of articulation, and over-exaggerate production of each sound in the words.

   FOUR GLIDES
   - wack, lack, yack, rack
   - woo, Lou, you, Roo
   - whap, lap, yap, rap

- wet, let, yet, Rhett
- wham, lamb, yam, Ram
- week, leek, yeek!, reek
- whip, lip, yip, rip
- whoa, low, yoah!, row
- way, lay, yeah!, ray
- ways, laze, yeahs!, raze
- whack, lack, yack, rack

THREE GLIDES
- why, lie, rye
- weed, lead, read
- wait, late, rate
- wake, lake, rake
- wade, laid, raid
- wed, led, red
- weep, leap, reap
- woes, lows, rose
- womb, loom, room
- white, light, right
- wick, lick, Rick
- wise, lies, rise
- wide, lied, ride
- wife, life, rife
- went, lent, rent
- wane, lain, rain
- wag, lag, rag
- wind, lined, rind
- west, lest, rest

W AND R
- what, rut
- wound, round
- woof!, roof
- whisk, risk
- wing, ring
- wince, rinse
- wipe, ripe
- witch, rich
- whiff, riff
- wig, rig
- wave, rave
- waft, raft
- one, run

L AND R
- lug, rug
- look, rook
- lush, rush
- lock, rock
- lice, rice
- leaf, reef
- load, road
- lot, rot
- loot, root
- loam, roam
- lobe, robe
- lone, Rhone
- lid, rid
- lift, rift
- like, Reich
- leach, reach
- law, raw
- lash, rash
- lace, race

4. Practice one-syllable words that contain both R and L. Produce these as if they had three syllables by treating R, L and the vowel as if they were their own syllables. Gradually blend the sounds together to make a smooth word. Make sure the distinct oral position and acoustic quality of each glide is honored. Focus on the sound of the glide that occurs between them. Do not reward the client if he adds extra sound to the transition phase between R and L. Gradually shorten the transitions to make a single word.

PRACTICE WORDS	PRONOUNCED
real	R-Ee-L
role	R-Oh-L
rile	R-I-L
rule	R-Oo-L
rail	R-A-L
lear	L-Ee-R
lair	L-A-R
lure	L-Oo-R

5. Practice multisyllabic words with both L and R. Produce L and R as their own syllables. Make sure the distinct oral position and acoustic quality of each glide is honored. Focus on the sound of the glide that occurs between them. Do not reward

the client if he adds extra sound to the transition phase between R and L. Gradually shorten the transitions to make a single word.

PRACTICE WORDS	PRONOUNCED
really	R-Ee-L-Ee
rolltop	R-Oh-L-Top
calendar	Ca-L-En-D-er
particle	Pah-R-TiK-L

6. Practice more words and phrases with R and L. Continue to separate R and L into their own syllables at first, and gradually blend the sounds together with mature transitions. Make sure that the distinct oral position and acoustic quality of each glide is honored. Focus on the sound of the glide that occurs between them. Do not reward the client if he adds extra sound to the transition phase between R and L. Again, gradually shorten the transitions to make a single word.

relay	relapse	relate	relook
religion	religious	relation	releasing
relax	relief	relieve	relinquish
relocate	release	relent	relentless
reliable	reliance	relief pitcher	relearn
relight	reload	relative	relativity
relegate	relevant	relic	roll
role	rolling	rollback	roll bar
roller skate	roller derby	roll bar	roll call
roller	roller rink	rolling pin	Rolex
roll-on	rollover	roll top	roly poly
roller coaster	rule	ruler	ruling
rule of law	ruling class	as a rule	rule of thumb
rule in	rule out		

7. Conjugate verbs that contain both R and L. For example, conjugate *to rule*. Practice these verb phrases alone and embedded in full sentences. Embed the phrase *cannot rule* into the sentence "The king cannot rule now." Avoid other R words in these utterances.

am ruling	am not ruling	
are ruling	are not ruling	aren't ruling
do rule	do not rule	don't rule
did rule	did not rule	didn't rule
can rule	can not rule	can't rule
will rule	will not rule	won't rule
could rule	could not rule	couldn't rule

would rule	would not rule	wouldn't rule
should rule	should not rule	shouldn't rule
might rule	might not rule	mightn't rule
could have ruled	could not have ruled	couldn't have ruled
should have ruled	should not have ruled	shouldn't have ruled
would have ruled	would not have ruled	wouldn't have ruled
might have ruled	might not have ruled	mightn't have ruled

Read Aloud

Reading aloud with correct R sounds can only be done once the client has learned to isolate the R sound and he has good control over it. This is a big leap forward in R training and a good transition to conversation. R occurs in random phonetic patterns in a written passage. Correct productions will require the ability to adapt to any and all on-glide and off-glide transitions. Further, oral reading requires that a client learn to recognize and prepare for the production of R while his mind also is processing the ideas of the written material. For many clients, reading aloud with correct R sounds is the final stage before complete mastery of the sound in isolation. The following tips are provided:

1. Select reading material that fits the client's reading level. Have the client bring his classroom reading as a way to discover his level without engaging in formal testing. Select other reading material that matches his skill level. Talk to his parents or teacher about his level.
2. Have the client scan the written material for R's before embarking on the reading. Consider highlighting the R words or underlining. Make photocopies of reading material that comes from books so that markings can be made.
3. Practice the R words included in the written material before doing the actual reading.
4. Assign reading aloud as homework once the client's skill is good in the treatment room.
5. Use the client's textbooks as practice reading material. In this way, R words that are important for specific teaching units can be rehearsed.
6. Make this work fun by seeking out humorous and excellent reading material. The easier Dr. Seuss books work great for beginning readers. Ask your local librarian or the classroom teacher for advice on good reads that capture the client's imagination and interests. Have the client bring in what he wants to read, and rehearse the important R words with him. Reading books the client loves enhances the therapeutic process. For example, a client who is fascinated by the Harry Potter books will delight in having an adult who is ready to help him learn to pronounce the unusual and amusing names of the characters.
7. Use the adolescent client's favorite recording artists as sources of reading material for R-word practice. Lyrics often are printed on CD jackets. If not, clients can investigate them on Internet sites and fan magazines. Although sometimes objectionable, the lyrics of popular songs comprise the poetry of today's youth. Many

young people are strongly attached to them as representations of their personal life experiences and opinions about life in general. These words can be a powerful way to build rapport with your adolescent and pre-adolescent clients. Watch out for violent and sexually explicit lyrics! Leave it up to the client to select pieces that he likes but that avoid these references. Teach him to edit out inappropriate language.

8. Students in religious training can use those texts as a source of reading material. Often these students have daily devotions or prayers that are recited. Practice for the week can be the correct reading or recitation of these required passages. Most parents appreciate other adults who are willing to address this material with their child. However, it is always wise to get at least verbal permission beforehand. Let the parents know you will not be teaching the content of the material, but merely helping the student apply his speech techniques into the oral material.

Use Negative Practice

Negative practice is an excellent tool to use during the later stages of therapy. It entails the purposeful misarticulation of the target phoneme. Hold off until the client can produce R with a high degree of consistent accuracy. Most clients can produce their own incorrect R any time during the course of treatment. However, during the final stages of treatment, a great number lose this ability. Suddenly, they discover that they cannot remember how to say R wrong. This is an excellent sign of progress! Realizing this is an outstanding way for the client to understand how far he has progressed in treatment. The client may have to relearn how to say the phoneme the old way. A client who can produce both the old and the new R should practice words alternately one way and then the other. This solidifies the new pronunciations as he comes to realize that the old way actually sounds wrong.

Spontaneous Speech

The ability to engage in real conversation using correct R sounds at all times is a tremendous feat if compared to the client's humble beginnings. Dialogue with correct R sounds represents the final stage of therapy. The following guidelines are suggested:

1. *R as Subject:* Early conversations should be about R itself. This keeps the client's mind on R while he is talking spontaneously. Talk about R words that continue to plague him. Review the process he has been through. Ask him with whom he has been using his new R sound, and discuss their reaction to it.
2. *Key Words:* Use key words to begin conversational work early in the treatment program. For example, once a client can produce his first cornerstone word, conversation can place emphasis on that word. He can practice using the word a great number of times. Ignore the other R's that occur during the conversation.
3. *Other Topics:* Spontaneous conversation can drift away from R and key words to any subject.
4. *Monologue:* Utilize the monologue to practice R. Ask the client to speak on a particular topic and let him know that you will be monitoring his speech. "Tell me

about the field trip you went on last week. Tell me everything carefully, and try to say each R correctly."

5. *Excited Feedback:* Sometimes we can treat errors in extemporaneous speaking excitedly and directly. We can stop our client mid-utterance with a robust, "Stop! Stop! Stop!" complete with flailing arms and excited facial expressions. The word in error can be reviewed and practiced. Then it can be practiced in a phrase or sentence appropriate to the monologue.

6. *Gentle Feedback:* Other times, treat spontaneous errors in monologue gently. For example, we can sit quietly until the client finishes his comment. Then we can ask, "Did you hear the error you made on the word? . . ." The word can be rehearsed alone and then re-embedded into a phrase or sentence.

7. *Message Confusion:* The only reason for clients to change their R pronunciation is for them to recognize that they are not being understood when they say R wrong. Conversational speech is a good time to focus in this area. Indicate to the client that you cannot understand him if he mispronounces. For example, a client might be talking about cars. The therapist can simply respond to the client as if he was talking about cows. "You want to own a red cow some day? I never saw one of those." These obtuse responses usually are quite humorous. They will lighten the client's feelings about making mistakes and encourage him to try harder to make the sounds correctly. Watch out! The client may enjoy your odd comments so much he will continue to make the phoneme incorrectly. That's okay. It's great negative practice.

8. *Signals:* Use a signal to reinforce good and bad R sounds that occur during your client's monologues and dialogues. For example, we can say "mhmmm," "yes" or, "good" quietly and nod while the client says each word with a good R. Or we can give thumbs up with each correct R. Sometimes we brighten our faces with each good R and darken them with bad ones. Style of response at this level of treatment comes from the personality of the therapist and the rapport she has established with the client. Keep in mind that students are not to be shamed with such feedback; they are to be instructed by it. Be clear with your signals and avoid unclear feedback that confuses the client and prolongs his training.

9. *Failure in Conversation:* Clients who are completely unable to maintain correct R sounds in monologues or dialogues are not ready to monitor their R sounds while speaking extemporaneously. Retreat to earlier levels of training.

Schedule Spontaneous Conversation Outside of Treatment

To ensure success, conversation often must extend outside of the therapy room. These methods differ depending upon work setting. At school, a brief, two-minute conversation in the hall between classes might be arranged. In private practice, a ten-minute telephone call midweek can do the trick. Use your imagination and break free of any preconceived notions about when and where therapy should occur for this aspect of treatment. During these final stages of therapy, two five-minute chats on the playground can be at least as valuable as any thirty-minute session in your therapy room.

Robert

The story of Robert is an appropriate one with which to end this chapter. Robert came to me at the age of nine after having been enrolled in R therapy for two years. In his prior therapy, Robert had been asked to practice a wide variety of R words in uncontrolled phonetic environments. But he could not produce even a single R correctly. And his oral-motor skills were poorly developed. Other phonemes had been in error earlier. There was still distortion on a few consonants and many vowels.

We began our therapy together by dropping the work on words and concentrating on more fundamental skills. Several months were spent training the tongue and jaw to move better. We worked on listening to and producing the vowels and L. I trained Robert's tongue to curl up and back in the classic Tip R position by using the techniques outlined in chapter 7. Together, this work helped Robert's cornerstone R to emerge in the vocalic position after Ah.

At least three months were spent solidifying this cornerstone sound. Robert had great difficulty saying it consistently. I taught him to say "Ah-R" by opening the mouth very wide for Ah, and then pressing the tongue tip up against the palate at the palatal notch for R. Although I knew that Robert could not continue to use this position forever, placing the tip against the palate at least allowed for a consistent true sound to become habituated. Robert began to discriminate true R, and his productions of this cornerstone sound became more consistent.

With his cornerstone sound at the ready, Robert systematically marched through each and every step outlined in this and the prior chapter. He worked on modifications of the cornerstone by adding other phonemes and syllables to it. We constructed practice lists of words, phrases and sentences for him to rehearse at home. He babbled with the cornerstone sound, and we built vowel charts with R for transition practice. He had to learn to suppress the inappropriate sounds he added to the off-glide. When he was ready, he learned to produce R next to adjacent consonants in blends by adding a schwa between the consonants and R. Robert's auditory discrimination of R developed well throughout this process.

After six months of training, Robert was in the final stages. He was able to perform all the ascribed lessons, and R had established itself at an 80 percent success rate in rapid conversational speech. But this was the R he had learned with the tongue tip placed against the palate at the palatal notch. There was a regular little flapping sound that was still heard in rapid conversational speech.

The high level at which R was appearing in conversation suggested that we reduce our schedule to biweekly treatment. During this period, I introduced Robert to the idea that R is actually made with the tip curled back but not touching the palate. His eyes bugged out when he first heard this. Not touching the roof of the mouth! This was a new idea for him. We had made the oral-motor pattern of his cornerstone sound and its transition movement rock solid. Therefore, Robert was able to produce R correctly without touching the palate on his first try, and he was able to make the sound consistently throughout that first session.

Robert was very pleased with his success, as he should have been. The idea arose that we could meet every three weeks. I agreed it would be good to reinforce his willingness to work more on his own. Robert had a wealth of practice material to review at home, and now he could discriminate his own correct and incorrect R sounds at will. Robert also was motivated to practice because he had had so much success in these six months. It was fun, interesting and easy!

During the eighth month, I noted a special change in Robert's production of R that assured me he would be completely successful even if treatment ended that day. His Tip R began to change into a Back R! This development demonstrated to me that not only had Robert learned to produce a great R, his oral-motor skills had improved significantly. Robert was beginning to use appropriate jaw stability and back-lateral tongue stability throughout all his speaking tasks. In my experience, a newly learned R never deteriorates once these oral-motor skills emerge.

Robert is still on my caseload, but soon he will drop to once per month. Then once per quarter, twice per year, and one follow-up a year later. Even though he is not quite finished, he has succeeded because R is present in his rapid conversational speech. His success has come as the result of determined plodding through a systematic training program that combined traditional articulation and oral-motor work to establish each and every stage of treatment. His auditory discrimination skills were advanced throughout the oral-motor facilitation exercises. At the beginning of our work together, Robert was considered a difficult client who was failing because he could not produce an R sound. Now he has become an easy client who is going to breeze through the rest of his program.

~ Summary ~

- *Transitioning* is the ability to on-glide and off-glide around the apex of R production. Transition work is the mountain of oral-motor work to be learned by difficult clients. This practice is most effective when organized around the vowels.

- Vowel transition work is organized around the five basic vowels learned by most students—A, E, I, O and U. These are used to represent all the vowels transcribed for the English language.

- Clients are taught to transition between their cornerstone R sound and other vowels. We begin with the identical vowel and then expand our work to include all the vowels.

- Transitions are used as the foundation of phrases and sentences in order to create a huge set of utterances with which to practice vocalic and consonantal transitions.

- Clients learn to move fluidly and rhythmically with repetitions of vowel transitions to and from R. Beat and rhythm properties of these syllables is stressed.

- Rate of speech is brought up to normal after accuracy has reached perfection at a slow pace.

- Rate of production is increased so that clients will come to recognize their personal speed limits. Clients are taught to adjust rate under the demands of various conversational speech situations.

- Most clients need specific work on R clusters. Many of these cluster patterns will be reflected in the client's personal set of "The Hardest Words in the World." R clusters reflect a variety of oral-motor patterns, and they are trained in various ways.

- Most clients will need special work on words that contain both R and L. We begin with simultaneous work on all the glides—W, L, Y and R—early in treatment to compare and contrast them.

- The ultimate key to successful R therapy lies in a client's ability to produce R in isolation, i.e., to articulate at the apex of R movement alone. With this skill a client can sound out any word with R.

- Reading aloud brings a client's newly generalized R into more difficult expressive speech tasks. Early reading should be slow. Add speed as accuracy develops.

- The final work of R therapy is to engage in spontaneous conversational speech using correct R sounds. This is done in monologue and dialogue, and in structured and unstructured ways inside and outside of the treatment room.

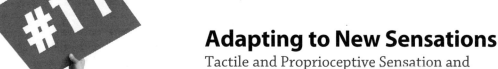

Adapting to New Sensations
Tactile and Proprioceptive Sensation and
New Phoneme Acceptance

Our discussion of treatment has focused on achieving a correct R from the first cornerstone sound to unstructured conversation outside of the therapy room. That is the meat and potatoes of R therapy. Now it is time to discuss the dessert, including the vibrotactile experience of R production. We'll keep it short and simple, just like the work itself.

Tactile and Proprioceptive Sensations

It is difficult to adjust to the physical changes involved in acquiring a new R phoneme. In fact, a change to any habitual movement pattern is difficult to make and slow to habituate. New movements feel awkward, uncomfortable, irritating and simply wrong. Consider the use of chopsticks. A person who grows up using a fork can have great trouble learning to use chopsticks. This is not because it is hard to use chopsticks. After all, millions of little children around the world use chopsticks with great skill every day. But when a person has spent most of life without them, simply holding chopsticks feels awkward. It requires coordinated hand and finger movements that have not been developed. It takes time to get the feel, and even longer before it seems normal to use them. This is true even when we have mature hand and finger control. Everything in us shouts, "I can't do this! It was easier the other way!" This is how most of our clients feel when they are learning to reposition the oral mechanism for a correct R sound. There is a natural tendency to resist.

Most readers understand that new movements practiced frequently can become habituated and comfortable over time. A fork feels normal if you always use it, but after using chopsticks for some time, chopsticks feel normal too. Likewise, the more frequently a client with a misarticulated R practices his new correct R sound, the more quickly he will adapt to these new sensations and accept them as normal. Our clients are being asked to acclimate to oral-movement patterns that are new and strange. The new R feels uncomfortable to them even if they have well-developed oral-motor skills. Our job throughout the process of treatment is to help them reverse this point of view.

We can feel the sound of R through two basic sensory channels: the *tactile* and *proprioceptive* systems. The proprioceptive, or *position sense,* allows us to perceive the movements made by our jaw, lips and tongue as we on-glide and off-glide to attain a phoneme's target position. These sensations arise from the contraction of muscles and the bending of joints. A correct R feels different than an incorrect one. The muscles and joints are picking up different movement data. Proprioception also allows us to feel both strength and fatigue in muscles. Many patients report that their jaws ache and their tongues get tired while learning a new R sound. This is because they are exercising oral movements in ways they never did before. Just like learning to use chopsticks, these new movements feel awkward and the muscles fatigue easily for a while.

The second way we feel R is through the tactile system. The production of an R is not like that of other phonemes with touching of lips, tongue and palate. The production of R requires little articulation other than the stability provided by the back-lateral margins of the tongue. R hangs out in the empty void of the oral cavity. Because of this, the tactile experience during production of R is a *vibrotactile sensation.* Think of it like this: Voice is sound, sound is vibration, and vibration is sensed with tactile receptors. The tactile receptors for sound production are located in the skin of the chest, throat, larynx, pharynx, oropharynx, palate, sinuses, head, inner and outer cheeks, lips, face and nose. The neurological end receptors in these areas are stimulated when the skin, muscles and bones near them absorb sound vibration. Every phoneme has a distinct feel picked up by the tactile system, just as each has a unique sound picked up by the auditory system. Both are the result of vibration produced at the larynx and resonating throughout the oral mechanism. A misarticulation of R feels different than a correct production because of the intensity and location of their vibrations.

The following two experiments will help the reader understand the vibrotactile element of sound production.

EXERCISE 11.1
EXPERIENCE THE VIBROTACTILE SENSATION OF SOUND

TRAIN YOURSELF TO ATTEND TO THE VIBROTACTILE SENSATIONS GENERATED BY PHONEMES BY THINKING ABOUT WHAT YOU FEEL IN YOUR CHEST, NECK, THROAT, PHARYNX, MOUTH, FACE, NOSE AND HEAD AS YOU PRODUCE SOUND. SAY EACH OF THE FOLLOWING SOUNDS ALOUD. STRETCH OUT EACH SOUND BY PROLONGING IT. PAY CLOSE ATTENTION TO THE SENSATION OF VIBRATION GENERATED BY EACH ONE.

"EE" "OO" "AH"   "OH"
"M"   "N"   "NG" "ER"
"Z"   "S"   "V"   "F"

Do you feel vibration with each sound produced? Do you feel a different amount or strength of vibration for each sound and how vibration is focused in a different place for each? Prolong each sound again and answer these specific questions:

- Do you feel the way M brings the focus of vibration to the front of the mouth, nose and lips?
- Do you feel the way N brings the focus of vibration inside the mouth?
- Do you feel how Ng brings the focus of vibration even further back to the oropharyngeal and back nasal areas?
- Do you feel the strong sense of vibration in the lips on Oo?
- Do you feel how Ah produces more sensation in the throat?
- Do you feel a strong vibration on Z and V?
- Do you feel a different type of vibration produced on the voiceless sounds S and F?

EXERCISE 11.2
Feel the vibrotactile sensation of various R productions

Train yourself to perceive the tactile differences between correct R and some of its misarticulations.

- Prolong a Tip R sound and focus on the vibratory sensations.
- Prolong a Back R and feel its vibrotactile sensations.
- Prolong R's with various distortions and feel the differences in the vibrotactile experiences. Compare them with the correct sounds.
- Prolong a W instead of R and feel the shift in vibration to the lips.
- Prolong a hypernasal R and notice the focus of vibration in the nasal cavities.

The vibrotactile sensations that differentiate one R sound from another are quite subtle. You may even have difficulty perceiving them in the experiments above. These differences are significant in therapy. They differentiate the feelings of abnormal productions in the minds of our clients. Unconciously, our clients think the old way of saying R is the way it should feel. Our persistent efforts to reposition the jaw, lips and tongue to achieve a better R will be undermined by the clients desire to re-create his old vibrotactile experience.

Successful R therapy should include activities that help a client reject the habitual feelings that comprise his incorrect R sound and accept the new sensations as his own. This work is subtle, like the sensations themselves. The work also can be emotional when a client clings to familiar patterns because he is afraid to take a new direction.

A tactile and proprioceptive focus requires almost no extra time or planning for R therapy. It's mostly comprised of the comments we make and the attitude we adopt as we progress through R therapy. The suggestions made below are presented in no specific order. It is recommended that these ideas be included intermittently throughout the long course of treatment.

Integrate Proprioceptive Experiences into Treatment
Take time to note the aches and pains of new movement learning. Open this topic by describing your own experience. "Wow. My tongue is getting tired from all this work." Or, "My jaw is beginning to ache. Is yours?" Allow moments of rest during intense oral-motor work. Encourage the client to rub his masseters to relax and rejuvenate his jaw. Let him sit quietly for a few minutes to rest overworked tongue muscles. Give him a drink of cool water or juice to refresh the mouth. Have tiny snacks at the ready for simple oral breaks. Talk on another subject for a moment. Or make sympathetic comments like, "It's hard to stretch the tongue back that far." Ensure the client that it will become easier. Make analogies to learning other physical skills. For example, many children experience hand cramps when learning to write. Help him see that those types of muscle aches diminish over time.

Talk About Vibrotactile Sensations
Draw the client's attention to the vibrotactile sensation of sound production. Begin by pointing out widely divergent sound sensations, and move gradually toward sounds that feel similar. The nasal consonants—M, N and Ng—are the easiest sounds to notice the vibrotactile element of sound production. One can feel these sounds vibrate throughout the oral and nasal cavities. For example, ask the client to prolong the M sound, and ask him to use his hands and fingers to feel the vibration on his lips and nose. Repeat this process with the other nasals. Compare and contrast the vibrotactile sensations of the nasals one to another, then to other sounds, and then to R. Use vocabulary that draws the client's attention to the vibratory sensations in the chest, throat, head, palate, lips nose and face. "Do you feel the vibrations of that sound? I feel it in my nose [lips/throat/throughout my face]. What do you feel? Where do you feel it?"

Assign specific vocabulary for the client to use in his explanations. Vibration can feel bumpy, tickly, or "buzzy like a bee." Give a specific title to these sensations such as the *buzzy feeling*, the *tickle in your nose*, or the *pressure in the back of your mouth*. Ask the client what he thinks the sensation should be called. An intellectual client may want to call it "vibration" while a class clown may want to call it "The Terrible Buzz." As long as you both know what you are talking about, shared vocabulary can become your little secret. It puts you and the child together in regard to this sound, which is great for building rapport.

Empathize about the New Unusual Sensation
Talk about the new tactile and proprioceptive sensations of R as they are realized. Empathize with the client about the unusual feel. Use words like *weird*, *wrong*, *awful* or *funny*. When

the client crinkles his nose after making the sound correctly, say, "It doesn't feel like R, does it? Pretty soon you won't even notice it anymore." The client may report that he doesn't like the new sensations. Assure him that he's not alone. "Lots of kids don't like it at first." Talk about other things the client may have learned that felt funny at first. Make an analogy to the process of acclimating to a new pair of shoes that felt stiff and awkward at first but comfortable over time.

Pair New Feelings with New Auditory Sensations
Make sure to link the new tactile and proprioceptive sensations to the the client's developing auditory discrimination of the correct sound, so that the two will become integrated and stored together.

In the learning process, new movements are cherished at the expense of sound quality. We have to tell a client not to be concerned about how his production sounds while learning. Then, when oral movements get better, we refocus their attention on the acoustic parameter. We can work back and forth from oral feeling to auditory sensation until the two meet together at the point of excellent R production.

Allow Emotions to Come Out
Tactile sensations are closely associated with emotions. Sometimes a client will become upset and cry when he realizes he can produce a correct R and feels it. The emotion is tied to years of frustration and hopelessness about ever learning a better way of saying R. He may have anger about his parents' expectations for his speech, or the teasing he may have received from other kids. He may be upset that a younger sibling learned R easily. He could be mad at a previous speech and language pathologist who could not help him with the sound. He even may be afraid to let go of his old R once he learns that he can make a better one.

Allow time in therapy for the client to air these feelings. Then move on. You do not have to psychoanalyze the revelation. You simply need to be there to listen. Short comments that show caring and empathy for the client's dilemma will suffice. "That boy should not have said that." Then wait for the client to express more.

Most clients will make another simple comment like, "Yeah, I hate that kid." Then they will be ready to move on. Clients usually don't want to spend time dwelling on hurt feelings. They want to get back on task and conquer their sound. Outside referrals to counseling will be appropriate on rare occasions. Therapists should use their best judgment about when such a referral may be necessary.

Make Errors to Compare Sensations
Once a new R sound is produced fairly consistently, draw the client's attention to his gradually diminishing errors, and even ask him to produce his old error on purpose as mentioned earlier. Some clients cannot produce their error sounds any more. This is a positive sign. If the client can make the error sound, however, this is an excellent time to work back and forth from good sound to error sound. Compare and contrast the way the two sound and feel. Talk about how the old sound is the one that is now starting to feel

funny. Use this time to praise the client lavishly for his success. When an error is produced, say, "What did you think about that one? Did it feel the same?" Then instruct him to try again, "Try to make it feel like the correct one." Don't engage in this work if producing the error sound causes the client to slip back into old habits. Wait a while, and drop it altogether if it proves too problematic.

Notice Lingual Tension

A client becomes highly aware of his tongue and its movements over time in R therapy. As this skill emerges, we can begin to focus his attention on the feeling of tension in the tongue. The client will begin to differentiate between the lax and the tense tongue. He also will be able to determine which part of his tongue is tense, which is lax and if the sides and the middle are up or down. These fine proprioceptive discriminations will help him take complete control over his production of R.

These skills usually are lacking in new clients. Do not expect them to respond to directions like, "Tighten up the middle of your tongue." Give these directions with direct stimulation early in therapy, and fade the stimulation over time as the client gains awareness and voluntary control of the actions.

~ *Summary* ~

- We feel the sound of R through two sensory channels: tactile and proprioception.

- Proprioceptive sensation allows us to feel the position of the jaw, lips and tongue during the on-glide, off-glide and target position for R.

- Tactile sensation allows us to feel the vibration of R as it resonates in the oral cavity.

- The sensation the client perceives for his incorrect R is that which he perceives as normal. Our efforts to reposition the jaw, lips and tongue will be undermined by the client's desire to re-create his old familiar tactile and proprioceptive experience.

- Successful R therapy includes activities that draw the client's attention to subtle tactile sensations of correct and incorrect sound production. R therapy helps them accept the new sensations as better and more appropriate.

- Drill a client's production of his corrected R sound so that the new tactile and proprioceptive sensations become ingrained in his mind along with the auditory sensation. These sensory experiences must be integrated and stored together.

- Empathize with the client about how the new way of producing R feels wrong or funny. Assure him that this new sensation is good, and inform him that the old sensations will be forgotten soon.

- Allow clients to express their pent up feelings about misarticulating R. Respond to these expressions with simple comments that show caring and empathy. Do not psychoanalyze these comments, but make referrals for counseling on those rare occasions when it is appropriate.

- Ask clients to alternate productions of both their old and new sounds on purpose to compare and contrast the way the two feel.

- Over time, clients learn to discriminate the precise tactile and proprioceptive sensations that occur as a result of a correct R production.

Capturing the Client's Attention

How to Engage, Inspire and Motivate Participation and Carryover

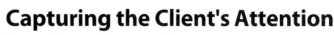

Motivation is one of the most challenging aspects of R therapy. Some clients enter the treatment room ready and willing to make this change. They want to work, they are ready to work, and nothing can derail them from their drive to learn R. We wish they were all like that. But let's face it: Many kids are completely unenthusiastic about attending weekly treatment to fix an R. Learning a correct R sound is not important to them, and weekly therapy is not their idea of fun. They see it as a necessary chore that promises to be boring and unrewarding. A bad attitude about treatment or an inability to fully understand the ramifications of what he is learning interferes with a client's drive for success. Therefore, we must capture the attention of the distracted client and focus the young client. We must motivate the unmotivated and encourage the discouraged. Ultimately, we must understand how to instill a willingness to learn in clients who simply don't care that they make better R sounds, as well as those who don't think they will ever be able to do so.

Motivating clients to succeed in R therapy is the third most important aspect of treatment. First and second are teaching the correct pronounciation of R and learning to on-glide and off-glide with other sounds. Motivating is that which draws clients into the learning process. It's what makes them want to say perfect R's all the time. We are not talking about games. Instead, we are referring to the ways we interact with clients so they develop a vested interest in this process.

There is no right or wrong way to encourage clients to participate actively in R therapy. In fact, there are as many techniques as there are therapists and clients. Every therapist and client contributes his own skill and interest in the subject. Personality and intellect play important roles. These factors mean that the content of individual therapy sessions varies from one client to another and from one session to the next. Peek in on any one R therapy session. It might look like a phonics lesson, a music class, a lecture, an oral-gymnastics workout, a spelling bee or a seemingly off-topic discussion about a family pet. Some sessions contain hundreds of sound productions. Others contain only one or two. Some sessions are spent digging through dictionaries for special words. Others are devoted to reading aloud with correct R sounds. The tone of individual sessions can range from serious to light and giggly. Counseling for the client or his parents can be a small part of periodic sessions or the main focus of an entire therapy program.

Of course, every therapist develops her own style. This chapter simply reflects the style I have developed over thirty years. Is this trivial? Absolutely not. This chapter will help readers understand the extent to which the logistics of treatment contribute mightily to the success of an R therapy program.

Design Approach by Chronological Age

Chronological age is a significant factor in designing an R therapy program. Articulation work with three-year-olds must be structured quite differently than that for thirteen-year-olds. The younger the client, the more the therapy will look like play. The older the client, the more the therapy will look like academic work. In addition, chronological age helps us determine the emotional demands of an R program. A strategy that matches the emotional needs of a client will help him focus on the task at hand. This is particularly important when it comes to pre-teens and teens.

The following guidelines are recommended for organizing R therapy by age to fit the intellectual and emotional capacity of clients. Designated age ranges should be viewed as fluid parameters, not rigid formulas. Professional judgment about the learning level of individual clients must help select every approach.

R THERAPY FOR TODDLERS

Although it is extremely rare that a therapist would enroll a toddler in R therapy, the subject does come up occasionally, especially regarding the offspring of speech and language pathologists as well as those clients with severe articulation disorder or phonological delay. Two-year-olds can engage in R therapy if it is oriented toward *vocal play*, a child's playful experimentation with his own vocal sound productions. The toddler is not able to focus his attention on any one particular sound too long. Therefore, a session devoted to R alone is almost impossible. Rather, the toddler will be entertained by the fascinating array of speech and non-speech sounds that can be made with the human mouth.

Successful R therapy for toddlers and other clients who function intellectually in this range should focus on producing a wide variety of sounds for the pure joy of their discovery, production and mastery. Repeat a wide range of sounds and oral positions. Toddlers are tricked into producing R through this vocal play and oral-motor experimentation. In fact, they can acquire R this way without realizing that they are working on it. The Tip R position is going to be the best position to train this group because it is easy to see and produce. Vocal play should include experimentation with five different aspects of sound production:

- *Environmental Sounds*: animals, motors, screeching tires, sirens, bells, whistles and so forth
- *Non-speech Vocalizations*: the sounds one makes while tongue-clicking, lip-smacking, kissing, chewing, swallowing, coughing, sneezing and so forth

- *Prosodic Features*: the loudness, pitch and intonation patterns of sounds, words, phrases and songs
- *Phonemes*: a wide variety of vowels, diphthongs and consonants including R
- *Oral Movements*: the playful discovery of a variety of facial and oral movements, especially tongue movements that bring the tongue tip up and back

R THERAPY FOR PRESCHOOLERS

R therapy can be quite successful with three- to five-year-old children, as well as those who function in that range. The younger and more immature clients in this range will need to continue the vocal play procedures. If imitation skill is good, a shift in general approach can occur as the client approaches the five-year mark and as he begins to show an interest in the alphabet. Therapy can move away from environmental and non-speech sounds and focus on the the sound of each letter in the alphabet. At first, a broad interest in all letters should dominate this play. Over time, the work can shift to R and its most similar-sounding letters, namely W, L and Y. It is best to keep therapy focused on all four of these sounds for a significant period of time. Early R can emerge out of a differentiation of these four sounds. The vowels and other sonorant phonemes, like M and N, also should be included. The Tip R is recommended for its ease in visibility and production by preschoolers.

An activity can be structured around magnetic alphabet letters. The therapist holds up one letter and says its name or sound. The child watches and then receives the letter to put up on a metal surface after he has imitated the therapist's model. The child believes he is playing a game. The therapist knows she is stimulating the client to pay close attention to the way phoneme are produced. Attention is drawn visually and by auditory means. Production of the letter and sound of R are embedded within the broader context of the whole alphabet. Over time, letter R can become the greater focus of such work, and the other sounds can be dropped.

Preschool children do not reject therapy when they think an adult is playing with them, when they believe they are the ones designing the activity, or when the teaching format is interesting. The preschool child must have an equal part in leading the activity. For example, pay careful attention to the way your preschool client naturally plays with alphabet letters. Devise procedures to match his play skill. If the child wants to toss the letters into a box instead of placing them on the metal surface, so be it. It does not matter what the activity is, so long as phonetic stimulation is included. Also, please remember that you are not testing the client's knowledge of the letters and their sounds. You are teaching. Therefore, tell him these names and sounds as often as possible for him to imitate.

Preschool children often clam up when they are put on the spot and expected to perform. When told to imitate a letter name or the sound it makes, they frequently refuse. Many therapists assume this means the child is not ready for articulation therapy. This is not true. The child is not ready for that approach, but he certainly is in a position to learn new sounds. Even without your intervention he will learn new sounds every day. A preschool child who refuses to do the work is showing you that the emotional demands of the approach are too high. Preschool children need to believe that we are playing with them, not working with them. Therefore, make your games easy, as if it were no big deal.

Show amusement in the sounds the letters make, and laugh when they are made in funny ways. If you model L, and the child says B, do not scorn him. Laugh with him at the funny way in which he changed the sound. The child is making a joke for you. If you show delight, he will do more. Over time, you and he will have a ball making all kinds of sounds together. Then you can slip in the R work along with the other easy sounds.

R THERAPY FOR THE YOUNG ELEMENTARY STUDENT

Once a child knows the alphabet and is beginning to sight read and sound out words, treatment for the misarticulated R can go straight to the phoneme itself. This will look like traditional articulation therapy. Most of these youngsters come willingly to therapy because it is something new and it offers the personalized attention of another adult. Though willing, the younger or immature elementary client may have no idea why he is coming to your room. When asked why they come, many answer "to play games or draw pictures." These young students should be told that they are coming to therapy to learn how to say R correctly. Their minds must be directed to the topic.

Review the alphabet so that the elementary client can gain a general understanding of how the R sound fits into the overall scheme of sounds in the English language. Early in treatment, focus should be placed on W, L, Y and R so that the client can compare and contrast these four similar-sounding phonemes. Many clients will have some trouble producing L correctly, as well. Teach L and R together for a while to give the client an opportunity to compare them. Talk about how R should sound. Written words can be the focus of work throughout treatment. But remember to write large for young readers. And although the Tip R or the Back R can be stimulated, the Tip R will continue to be the easiest in this age range.

Most elementary age children become self-conscious of their error some time during this period due to comments made by others outside of therapy. These students can be told that although R is difficult, they can and will learn it. These children can be told they are not alone and that R is "the hardest letter of all." Although most elementary children attend R therapy willingly, that begins to change as they become preteens.

R THERAPY FOR 'TWEENS

By eleven or twelve years of age, most clients are fully aware they cannot say R. Pre-teens begin to fall prey to group pressure, and they want to be the same as everyone else in their peer group. Therefore, if they believe that saying an R incorrectly makes them stand out, they will come to therapy willingly. However, if they believe that none of their friends notice the error and that going to therapy is what will make them stand out, then they will reject it. This is especially true if they must be pulled out of regular classes to go to the speech room at school.

'Tweens often are burning with energy. They are driven to try anything and everything. They want immediate action their own way. The slow pace of articulation therapy can be impossible for them to bear. Pre-teens must believe that they are not wasting their time in working with us. I find it very helpful to show them that I understand this. "I wish you didn't have to come." Then I assure them that I know exactly how to help them make a correct R. Sometimes, I even tell them that I am the "best R teacher" in town. 'Tweens must be told that they do not know how to learn R on their own and that they need help.

Many pre-teens will develop a commitment to R therapy when we model back to them the way they sound. These children can be quite shocked to hear it. They really do not understand how bad they sound until they hear it coming from another person. We talked about this technique earlier when we discussed imitation of the client to help us understand his error and as a way to help him discriminate his own error. Now we are talking about using the echoing technique to help the client connect emotionally to how he sounds. I may begin suddenly to talk on any subject using a perfect imitation of a client's sound. They often respond by saying something like, "I don't sound like *that*, do I?" This is not meant to be cruel. It is meant to open up the child's conscious awareness of what he is doing. Upon seeing and hearing this, many make a decision to begin therapy immediatlely!

Another way to approach this is to write a word like *car* with bold letters on a piece of paper. Ask the client to say the word aloud. Model his distortion back to him by saying, "You said . . . . Most people say . . . ." and say the target word with correct articulation. Repeat this example several times with the same word and with other R words. Work slowly to allow time for the idea to sink in. Carefully observe the client's face so you will be sensitive to that moment the truth dawns. When you see the wheels turning inside his head, you know he is realizing the truth about his own R. Allow him time to respond. Ask, "What do you think?" or, "What do you hear?" Help him get past his own denial.

'Tweens will need to learn some patience in R therapy. They must be told that R may not be said correctly the first day or the first month. They have to be told that the only way they will learn R is to do exactly what you tell them to do. They need to understand that there are some mouth exercises that will help. If they do them, they will learn R soon. They are told that they are not simply going to practice saying R words over and over again. They are going to learn tiny steps that will teach them the R.

Most pre-teens arrive at a decision to enter therapy when their focus becomes future directed. Therefore, I ask these children to think about what they want to do when they grow up. Then I try to help them see how good speech will be a part of their plan. I also ask them to think about how they want boys or girls to think about them in middle school, junior high or high school. By then, the other students will notice the problem.

I believe that 'tweens who cannot get with the program must be given the option to quit. This is not simply because I want stubborn children off my caseload—although that is tempting. Therapy will fail without their active participation and cooperation. This does not mean coming to the therapy room every week on time because the parents or the teacher made them. It means dropping the resistant attitude and getting to work. I tell my clients this without being mean. In straightforward terms they can understand, I say, "If you want to work on your R now, we can do it. If you don't want to work on it and if you won't do the work, then there is no reason for us to do this." If they choose not to come, I explain that I will contact them in six months or one year to see if they are ready. I let them know that when they make the decision to change their R, they will be able to do so and I will be there for them.

Some 'tweens do an about-face right when they hear such straight talk. The pleadings or stern talk of their parents may have been worth a rebellion, but straight talk from someone outside the family makes them think about this problem logically. This is good. Get them beyond their early experimentations with teenage rebellion by offering an opportunity to think through the problem and respond to it as an adult. When given this choice, many respond enthusiastically. One tough eleven-year-old boy recently told me he was going to be a professional basketball player and, therefore, did not need to say his R sounds correctly. I said, "That's really cool! Being a professional basketball player would be so fun! If you're really good, you'll be interviewed on worldwide television. You won't mind talking in front of millions of people with a bad R?" I could see the wheels turning in his head as he pictured himself being interviewed in the locker room after the big game. He changed his mind that moment.

Of course, a few 'tweens and teens will need more time. Some of these kids like their incorrect R because they want to be different than the crowd. Others are still in denial. If more time is needed before the initiation of a therapy program, I instruct parents to back off from nagging their child about the problem. I tell them that it's not worth the fight. When the child is ready, he will do the work well. This is hard for some parents. They may need time to talk with you privately about their fears in waiting for therapy to commence. Many parents point out that they are afraid their child will be teased because of the incorrect R. I tell these parents that teasing may be exactly what the child needs to get him motivated. I tell them that when this occurs, they can say, "Well, just let me know when you want to work on that and we can go back to see Mrs. Marshalla." I may work out a plan with the family to help them handle this waiting period. For example, the parents may be instructed to ask the child about therapy no more than once a month. More will be viewed as nagging. Many parents will mark their calendars ahead for the specific days on which they can pose this question. I may tell the child that he should expect to hear this question, and that he is to answer it with a simple yes or no. I also tell the child and his parents to call any time he is ready to work, if that occurs in less than the assigned waiting period. In the meantime, I may give the child one or two simple oral-motor exercises. I tell him that if he does the assigned oral-motor exercise, therapy will go much more quickly once he gets started. He even may learn R on his own if he does it often enough. Then I teach him how to curl the tongue back for a Tip R, and I let him go.

For some kids, there are exceptions to this hands-off policy. Sometimes it is the parents who need the prodding. These parents are afraid to make their kids do what they need to do. The parents need to learn how to say, "No, it is time to do this work *now*." When to back off and when to push forward is difficult in all aspects of parenting. That is no different when it comes to R therapy. Whether he is enrolled now or later, most children eventually will learn R if given good treatment. I usually assure parents that therapy does not have to take place immediately. I ask them to think about what they would like their child to have learned by the time he turns 18. I suggest that some time between now and 18 is when he will learn R. This usually takes the pressure off and gives the parents and the child a chance to make a clear decision about the time of enrollment.

Another aspect of articulation therapy for pre-teens and teens has to do with gender. Put simply, some young male clients are tired of being told what to do by females. They see their moms and their teachers—mostly women—as trying to boss them around while they are trying to become men. At a certain point in their development, they must reject the strong influence of women in their lives in favor of male influences. Boys entering this natural maturing stage often do better with male therapists. They find that the intimate work of R and the emotional baggage that comes with it can be faced better with a male mentor. I try to honor this whenever I can by referring such boys out to male therapists in my community. This is easy in private practice. Unfortunately, assigning a particular male student to a male therapist often cannot be done in the public school. Referral to an outside source may be an option. Also, postponing therapy until the child moves up to the next school where a male therapist serves may be a solution.

Many speech and language pathologists use written contracts for 'tween and teen participation in R therapy. The contract references his willingness to participate, his promise to come to therapy regularly and on time, his agreement to do assignments, and so forth. Written contracts are especially useful for the school setting that limits the number of times a therapist can consult with parents. Written contracts are perhaps less necessary in the private sector since parents transport children and pay directly for services.

Privacy is another issue that plagues the pre-teen and teenage client. Adolescent clients need to understand that what goes on in the therapy room is private between the therapist and the client. This is easier to accomplish, of course, in individual therapy. In group therapy, the client has to have some assurance that what is said in the group stays there. This is one of the reasons I love private therapy for these clients. Private therapy affords an opportunity for clients to express the deeper issues of their articulation problems.

Sometimes 'tweens and teens want to sign up for two or three lessons to see how it goes before they are willing to commit to an entire process. This is an excellent option that usually results in enrollment once the client gets more familiar with the therapist and the therapy process.

R THERAPY WITH TEENS AND ADULTS

Some young teens respond with rebellion like the 'tweens described above. If so, they should be treated the same way. Mature teens and adult know they cannot say R, and they attend therapy because they want to learn it. Fixing the incorrect R is the only reason they come. Thus, therapy can commence with a direct approach to R and its pronunciation. Mature clients often are fascinated with phonics, which can become a theme in treatment. I try to wow them a little with my knowledge of phonetic transcription to pique their interest. General discussions on pronunciation, spelling, root words, other languages, accents, dialects, public speaking and other topics related to speech and language can enrich your discussions. Noticing speech errors by television journalists is an excellent way to help mature clients see the broader issues related to pronunciation. Some clients will benefit from reading parts of this book. Many mature clients will have certain goals in their desire to learn R. For example, high-school students may be looking forward to entering college with a correct R sound. College students may be anticipating their first job interview with good speech. Some students even may be considering linguistics, translation or speech pathology as career options. These aims should be included in therapy discussions. Adult clients who come to therapy for R are rare. Usually, these clients are highly motivated. They often have misconceptions about who is to blame and why they could never learn R in the first place. Discussion may include venting about past failures, parent pressure or previous teachers involved this endeavor.

Talk about R as a Subject unto Itself

Children who are of elementary age and older usually need information to help them see the big picture when it comes to mispronunciation of R. They need to see that R is a difficult sound to learn and that it is a common error. They are not the problem; R itself is. The ideas listed below help our clients settle into the process of articulation treatment for R. We can bring these ideas up all at once in the initial evaluation or treatment session, or we can bring them up throughout the long haul of therapy. Please realize that not all clients need to know all this information. These bits of information are selected for inclusion in R therapy when it is determined that they may be valuable.

THE CLIENT IS NOT ALONE

Teach your client that there are hundreds of thousands, perhaps millions, of children who have difficulty learning the North American English R sound. I usually do this by helping them realize that there are between one and ten children who cannot say R in every school in the entire country. That is a lot of kids. Help them recognize they probably know other children who cannot say R. You can leave these children's names out so that the discussion does not sound like gossip. Instead, refer to them by using phrases like "one boy I know" or "the kid I'm talking about." Help the client see that although he may be the only person in his family or his small group of friends who has this problem, there are thousands of people just like him who struggle with R.

R IS HARD TO LEARN

Inform your client that it is so hard to learn to say R that it usually is the last sound children learn to say correctly when they are learning speech. Some children learn R earlier, some later. Tell your client that he simply has not learned the last sound yet. Now is his time.

R IS RARE

Clients should be told that R is so hard to say that many languages do not even use it. For example Japanese has no R sound, and neither do many other Asian languages. Call the North American Standard English R "the hardest sound in the world." Talk about the difference between the French, Spanish and English R sounds. The French R is a voiced velar fricative, and the Spanish R is a voiced lingua-alveolar trill. Learn to produce these sounds yourself so you can demonstrate them for your client. Play around with these other R sounds with the client to see if he can produce them.

IT TAKES TIME TO LEARN R

Help your client see that it takes most children about one year to learn to say R perfectly. Help him see that the length of time necessary to change his R will depend upon him. Teach him that his speed in learning will depend upon how well he listens, how often he does the work, and how hard he tries. (Keep in mind that if the client is not succeeding a little bit every session, the problem lies not in the client but in your technique.)

THERAPIST AND CLIENT HAVE DIFFERENT ROLES

Inform your client that your job is to teach him the R sound and that his job is to follow your instructions. Inform him that you will assign activities that seem to make no sense. "You will have to trust that I know what I'm doing and that the things I ask you to do will help." Tell him that, in the end, he will see how every activity fits together and he will learn to say R perfectly.

SOME WORK IS EASY. SOME HARD

Teach your client that he can breeze his way through the easy work, but he must try very hard on the difficult activities. Help your client realize that he does not have to be shy about telling you the difficulty he is having. Encourage him to talk about the activities that are easy and hard. Tell him that the more he gives you this type of feedback, the more you can adjust your activities to fit his skills.

HELP CLIENTS FACE THE TRUTH

On occasion, it is necessary to tell a client that if he doesn't speak R well, some people will think that he is not smart enough to learn it or that he is not smart enough to get help for it. Help your client realize that it is worth a few months to learn R now so that he can avoid all this as he grows up.

Reward Client Performance

Except for the young client who can be tricked, the ability to say a correct R is the only prize worthy of finishing a treatment program. Our clients must discover how to care about their own speech, not because someone tells them they should care, but because they really do care. With the ability to produce a correct R comes the pride of accomplishment. It is the good feeling of knowing the people who care for you are pleased. It is relief that the problem is over. It is the control of managing a difficult task. A therapist in charge of an R program must design treatment to build this sense of internal reward by managing the external reward system.

The crux of behavior modification lies in the basic performance-reward paradigm. A reward is something given for merit. It is earned. Clients who engage in the work of R therapy should be rewarded for their efforts. A reward system contributes significantly to client motivation and success in the program. The purpose of a reward system is to get the client on track and to keep him there through the long haul of R therapy. Rewards need to be meaningful to the client. Therefore, we don't offer star stickers to clients who don't care, and we don't praise clients lavishly if it makes them uncomfortable. We must know our clients and discover the type of reward that will make a difference. Some kids crave tangible rewards, like stickers and stars, while others ignore them and respond much better if you tell them how great they are doing. The following ideas about reward procedures in R therapy are offered in no specific order.

TANGIBLE REWARDS

A tangible reward is an object given for good performance. Tangible rewards include stickers, stars, smily faces, small trinkets, candies and so forth. Tangible rewards have their place, but they will take clients only so far. No client will work through an entire articulation therapy program for sweets, stickers or smily faces drawn on paper. These things are fun and motivating for a little while, but once the child has received a few of them, they lose their appeal. Clients say, "So what if I earn another sticker" and, "I don't like that candy!" Still, tangible rewards can be an integral part of all aspects of R therapy. They are a nice way to keep things moving forward.

VERBAL PRAISE

Verbal praise is the most important form of reward in R therapy. It is the primary tool we have to build a client's desire to participate in treatment, and it is our main tool in shaping a client's understanding of the process. Therapists should stay away from nebulous verbal responses like "good job" or "good talking." Use more meaningful responses that instruct the client, "Perfect! You said that one exactly right." Or, "Good, you listened very carefully." Or, "Now your tongue is moving better!" Comments with content bring the purpose of therapy into focus. They teach clients what they are doing. They let them know in exact terms what is wanted.

IMMEDIATE REWARDS

Immediate rewards are those given on the spot. They reflect a client's performance on individual trials, and they reflect a client's performance that day. For example, when a client identifies an incorrect R spoken by the therapist, he is rewarded with a star immediately after his response. Or after a client participates well in a therapy session, he is rewarded with a positive statement to the parent who is waiting for him in the lobby. Different kinds of immediate rewards can be paired together. A therapist might draw a smily face on the client's paper while saying "Perfect!" in response to a production.

SHORT-TERM REWARDS

Short-term rewards are given to mark significant progress. They signal that the client is doing well although the end is still far off. For example, after six weeks of therapy, the therapist might write a short note to the parents. "Johnny is doing the best work he possibly can at this point of treatment. He cannot say the R sound yet. But he is doing everything I ask him to. He is working hard on the things that will make him able to say R soon." A note such as this can be written while the student watches. Sometimes I ask my clients what they would like me to say to their parents. Most kids give a specific idea, "Tell Mom I got to your room on time," or, "Tell them they shouldn't worry about my R sound." These insights into home life can add tremendous depth to an R therapy program.

TANGIBLE SHORT-TERM REWARDS

Short-term rewards also can be tangible items, like a pack of gum, a small toy or a new pen. Many therapists keep a treasure box full of small items children can choose. I buy these small items inexpensively at garage sales. I go late on Saturday afternoons, when I know families want to unload as much as possible. I usually pay a few dollars to take a whole box of toys off their hands. Then I sort through them at home and toss the ones that are no good. A treasure box is always ready for those special days when the client has earned a special treat. Treasure boxes full of reward trinkets can be purchased from many distributors of speech materials.

LONGTERM REWARDS

The longterm reward is a significant, tangible object or event selected by the child and given at the end of the program. It is one that the child would not otherwise receive, and it is purchased by the family. Most clients will not need a big reward at the end of R therapy. In fact, it is hoped that most clients will be so happy that they have finally learned to say R that they won't need one. But some clients need to have the promise of a longterm reward in order to sustain them until therapy is over. The longterm reward is discussed early in therapy but not given until the goal has been met. Longterm rewards might include a new bike, an opportunity to select the next family vacation or a trip to the local video arcade. Since longterm rewards are needless and expensive in most cases, they should not be brought up unnecessarily.

BRIBES

A bribe is something given beforehand to convince or cajole. But it isn't any good. For example, a candy bar can be given before therapy so a child will do his work. Because the candy is given beforehand, it will not be effective in motivating a child to work hard in R therapy. What will you do if the child quits after you have provided the bribe? Rewards given after good performance are more effective and will take the process further.

GIFTS

I like to give unexpected gifts occasionally to my clients. I might give a teen girl a little diary, or a young boy a toy car. These little pre-wrapped gifts can be kept handy for distribution during a surprise moment in treatment. Reserve them for that one time in the process of treatment when things are getting a little glum and the client is becoming despondent. Don't make the present a reward for good behavior, and certainly don't let it seem like a bribe. Make this a simple gesture to let the client know you like him. Also, consider doling out inexpensive holiday gifts to all the clients. The right little gift at the right time can help develop rapport and motivate participation.

Construct Timeframes

One of the greatest factors that contribute to a client's lack of motivation is ignorance about how long the process of therapy will take. We make a mistake to enroll R clients in treatment with no hint of its conclusion. It makes therapy seem like a life sentence. Take a hint from children's sports activities. Swimming and gymnastic classes are scheduled to run for a certain period of time. There is comfort in knowing that the classes will end on a certain date. Even sports like baseball and soccer have a season that ends at a certain predetermined date. Championship matches always drag these seasons out, but at least the families know generally when the season will be over. We should do this in R therapy. Clients can accept a treatment program more easily if they know when they can get out. They and their parents need to have a general idea about how long R therapy will take.

Most readers will think, *We never know how long a certain client's R program will take!* This is true, but we manage this by enrolling clients in a definitive period of time that is repeated if necessary. In private practice, we can schedule the client for three months of treatment with the understanding that we might extend it for another three months. In public school, a client can be scheduled for one trimester or one semester with the understanding that he might need an additional term afterward. A definitive timeframe allows all involved to settle into the schedule. It also incorporates an expectation of review at the end of each time period. A specific timeframe lets the client know when he might opt out if he's not ready or not committed. It also lets parents know that you are willing to end the process if that is appropriate. It's easier to end or postpone therapy when that possibility is discussed beforehand.

I usually tell my families that R therapy will takes at least two three-month periods, and sometimes more, depending upon the client. I ask families to commit to the first three-month session without expecting dramatic results. By the end of three months, it will become obvious whether or not the client is benefitting from this work. A decision can be made between parents, therapist and client to continue or not. Framing therapy is especially important in private practice when parents are paying directly for services. Three-month blocks of time are helpful.

Determining a timeframe for R therapy also involves consideration of other competing activities, such as sports, driver education, the birth of a sibling, or family vacations. R therapy is important and should be scheduled when other events and activities are not competing for the child's time. R therapy is not another activity that can be tagged on to the end of a busy week. Space in the schedule needs to be carved out during a time when the child will not be exhausted or distracted by competing activities. Therapy also needs to be scheduled during a time when many sessions will not be missed due to vacations. A problem in this regard is often seen in private practice. Parents often have good intentions about getting their child to speech therapy in the summer. They do not foresee how many times the client will have to miss treatment due to vacations, camps and the like. It is important to help parents take a realistic look at their family calendar to determine if beginning R therapy will be appropriate. Often, it becomes obvious that weekly therapy during the summer will not be consistent enough to make a real impact upon the client, and that therapy should be postponed until school starts in the fall. If parents insist on summer therapy, I make sure they understand that regular attendance is critical to a successful outcome.

Some of our R clients fail during the schoolyear because they simply do not have time to think about what they are learning in therapy. I recently saw a twelve-year-old girl who needed work on R and other phonemes. This girl was being driven one-hour (!) to and from private school every day. She received private reading and math tutoring several times a week after school. And she was seeing another speech and language pathologist on Saturdays to work on conversational language skills. When I asked what she liked to do when she had free time, she told me she had no free time. I told the mother that I could not consider putting her daughter on my schedule until she had a lighter load. The mother did not like my answer and just about stormed out of my office. I never heard from them again. I do feel a pang of guilt when I think about her, but I saw a look of relief on the child's face. Perhaps the only good thing I did for this client was to show her that the amount of work she was being expected to handle was unreasonable.

Finally, use a calendar to note the date treatment is initiated. Then use it to discuss how long the client has been in therapy and how much longer he may have to go. Count the weeks or number of sessions he has attended, and discuss the skills he has learned during that time. "On March 23rd, you could not say R at all. Now here, on June 16th, you can say R at the beginning of any word! In 12 weeks you have learned about half of what you need to learn." Specific information about what he has learned and how long it has taken him to learn it gives perspective to the process and deepens the client's commitment to it.

Take Tiny Steps

Each session of treatment should add only one or two tiny pieces to what has been accomplished. Leaping quickly to more advanced levels only causes distress as clients begin to practice things for which they are not ready. To the client and his family, it seems as if R should be learned quickly and easily. But R therapy often is not like that, especially with difficult clients. When we leap too quickly into more advanced work, we almost assure that the difficult client will fail. With tiny steps, clients practice only that which they can do well. We create the impression the work is easy. This is a boon to therapy. The greatest compliment we can receive when working with R clients is for them to exclaim, "This is so easy!" It means that our work increments are small enough for high levels of success.

For example, after a client learns to sequence R-Ah with you in a session, stop. He has learned one thing, and that is enough for the week. Practice that one skill a dozen times. Then demonstrate it for the parents if possible. Then ask the client to practice this one skill for homework five times a day that week. When the client comes back for the following session, review his work and praise him if he did it well. Then move on to a few words that begin with R-Ah such as *rock, rob, rod* and *Ron*. Have the client practice these four words several times. Add no more work to that session. Ask him to practice these four simple words once a day until he comes back.

There are many reasons why tiny steps work best for success. First, the client will have specific work to practice during the week, and he will have a small set to demonstrate for the family. A small set is easier to practice and to demonstrate for others. A small set can be memorized easily for extra practice at random times throughout the week. Tiny work increments also are easier to incorporate into conversational speech early in treatment. For example, after learning to say *Ron*, the client can begin to talk about a real or imaginary boy named *Ron*. He will have to speak slowly, but the basic work will be there. Minute steps like these assure better results than practicing random word lists. Taking tiny steps is the only way some clients master their R sound.

There will be times when a client makes huge gains rapidly. Tiny steps will only frustrate them. One day, Aaron learned a perfect R after months struggling to get his tongue in the right position. He finally got the right sound and was thrilled. I could not stop him from trying all kinds of words during that session, most of which he was not ready for. But this client needed to see for himself what he could do once he got the sound. After about twenty minutes of trying this word and that, Aaron looked to me for guidance. I began to make a list of the words he was ready for and could practice at home. I could see that he felt defeated by such a small list of words, so I told him that he could feel free to experiment with all kinds of words at home that week, as long as he kept up his practice on our short list. Aaron came back the following week having mastered much more than our list. We used that session to explore all that he could do. We made a somewhat longer list for the next week, but again he was told to experiment. By the third week after having learned his cornerstone R, I could not hold him back. Aaron was ready to fly! We moved immediately into reading because Aaron was ready to tackle any and all words with R.

Create an Old-Fashioned Speech Binder

Nothing helps solidify an articulation program more than creating an old-fashioned speech binder. "Ho-hum!" But wait! For many years I too thought this was a corny idea. In the past six years, however, I have begun to use speech binders regularly. I have realized numerous benefits. A binder that grows by a few pages each week becomes a permanent record of all the work the client does in articulation therapy. It is a wonderful way to review material, a fantastic way to keep parents informed about treatment, and an amazing way for the client to track his progress. The ability to see what is being accomplishing week after week helps motivate clients to keep going until the end. The speech binder also is a great way for multiple therapists who are working with the same client to keep track of what each other is doing.

A speech binder can be a primary tool of motivation. One client, Alex, reached beyond page 100 in his speech binder before he was dismissed from R therapy. This six-year-old was proud of this collection of accomplished material. We talked about his binder as a book of 100 pages that he had written himself. The binder was his great motivator and the primary tool that his mother used to practice with him at home. His mother, Sharon, and her son's persistent work with his speech binder was the key to his final success on R.

The following suggestions are made regarding design and use of a speech binder.

- The speech binder is constructed with papers that are made in therapy sessions. One-inch, three-ring binders work best. They hold a lot of material and are easy to flip through and move work around in.
- Parents are asked to supply the child with the binder. This way they have a vested interest in keeping track of it at home. Keep a small supply of binders to give away for clients unable to purchase their own. Buy them in bulk to keep the price low.
- Place pages created in treatment directly in the binder from back to front, so the most recent work is always on the first page when the binder is opened. If a page

of special homework directions is needed, this goes in last during a session and becomes the front page.
- A client numbers each page as it goes in the binder so the numbering of the book ends up being backward. Kids get a kick out of this. Numbers are simply changed if pages are relocated.
- Use unlined white paper and colorful markers to make the pages. Keep a three-hole punch handy for the appropriate holes and immediate binding. Create a simple hole-punch-page-numbering ceremony to mark the conclusion of each session.
- Every piece of session work can be recorded in some fashion. The paper can be placed in the binder. Include all spontaneous pictures the client draws as well.
- Place special handwritten letters praising the client's performance in his binder for him to show to his parents. Draw simple charts to record progress. Make pages that list things the client has learned.
- Make pages of oral-motor exercises. Use words that the child can understand. Ask the client what words to use to explain these exercises so that he can remember how to do them at home. Draw simple pictures with bold lines to teach oral parts, positions and movements.
- Make word, phrase and sentence lists to practice in therapy sessions and at home.
- Date each page at the top so that you can always determine how long the client has been working on specific skills.
- Write checks or stars next to each item you review, and reward the child's achievement on specific activities by placing smily faces and stickers on the pages. Do so each time you review a page. Write "Very Good!" "Perfect!" or "Excellent!" on the top of each page he does exceptionally well. Some pages will end up with dozens of reward marks of various colors and shapes all over them. These pages look beautiful by the time you are done, and the client will be proud of this work.
- Taking binders to therapy and back home again is easy in private practice, where parents are carting their children to and from treatment. In public school, consider creating a section in the child's regular class binder for speech work.

Work pages created on the spot for the speech binder are something I love to do with my clients. I find that if I draw and write the information on the page as they watch, they are drawn into the process more than if we use pre-printed workbook pages. Handmade pages can be colorful and can use large lettering, simple drawings, lines, arrows, circles, boxes and other symbols to help clients understand their work. Handmade pages faithfully represent the detail of R work as we have outlined it in this book. Published workbook pages are included where appropriate. Photocopies of reading material also are included.

Engage the Mind to Ensure Carryover
A client's mind can wander in a thousand different directions if he is not stimulated to think about the work at hand in R therapy. Children of elementary age and older who are enrolled in R therapy should be stimulated to think about why they come to therapy. A

mind that is engaged in the process will create faster and more solid changes. A focused mind helps a client become more deeply committed to the process of change.

All the work we have discussed throughout this book has been designed to help focus the mind on R. But we can do even more when we ask certain questions designed to help the client think through his therapy experience. Specific questions force a client to think how speech relates to his life and the people with whom he communicates. For example, we might ask:

- "Why do you come here?"
- "What do we do here?"
- "What have you learned so far?"
- "What can you do with your new R?"
- "What can't you do yet?"
- "What do you want to learn today?"
- "What do you want to learn next week?"
- "How much longer do you think this will take?"
- "Why will it take that long?"
- "Who do you show these skills to?"
- "Have you used these skills with anyone at school?"
- "Can you use this skill in school this week?"
- "Have you used this skill on the telephone?"
- "Who could you show this skill to?"
- "Has your mom said anything about your speech yet?"
- "How do you know your speech is getting better?"

Easy questions, like the first one, can be asked right from the onset of treatment. More difficult ones, like the last one, are reserved until later. Usually a question or two like these are included every few sessions. Entire sessions can be devoted to these discussions, especially during the later stages of treatment. Therapists should not view discussions on these topics as a waste of time. Our clients need time to understand how to incorporate this work into their broad communication life. These discussions help assure carryover of skills into all aspects of conversational speech.

Examine Your Efficiency
Nothing destroys an R therapy program more than wasting time, and wasting time destroys motivation and commitment to the process. In my opinion, the greatest waste of time in R therapy is the board game. This occurs on two levels. First, time is lost setting up the game, tossing dice, spinning wheels, picking cards, moving pieces and arguing about rules. All these things drag out the process of R therapy. I began to think about this even as an undergraduate. I remember watching upper classmen using board games in therapy and asking myself, "Why don't they just get to work?" Time in therapy is special. None of it should be misused.

More importantly, the greatest trouble with board games in articulation therapy is that they take the client's focus off the sound of R and put it on the game. Most of the clients cannot organize their thoughts around two things at the same time. If they are thinking about R, then they cannot process the game. And if they think about the game, they cannot listen to what I have to say about R. The board game is far more interesting to most students than anything I have to say about R. Most clients in R therapy need to be helped to focus. Their attention needs to be captured to the exclusion of everything else. Board games often are not conducive to this.

However, there always are exceptions! Some clients can and do engage perfectly well with therapy around a board game. In fact, a game can draw certain clients into therapy when they otherwise would not be interested. Therapy is a balancing act. Some kids will not be able to handle board games, while others will need them. The trouble comes when we match kids and activities in the wrong way, or when we mix kids with different learning styles together in groups. If you use board games in therapy, make sure to ask yourself how much time is devoted to the game and how much is focused on R. You may discover that too much time is being tossed out the window by using games. If so, reduce the number of times you rely on them, and increase your attention to the process of learning R. Ultimately, our clients need to feel the reward of producing R itself, not in winning a board game.

Another time waster can be the sports activity, when clients produce sounds or words and then are rewarded by tossing a ball into a hoop, kicking a ball, fishing for toys or cards, etc. These are great activities to encourage drill practice at the sound, word, phrase or sentence level. They are a disaster when the client is first learning the sound, and especially if the client cannot integrate the play with the work. Take a good look at your therapy to determine if time is being focused on the activity to the exclusion of learning the sound.

Make Drill Work Interesting

We have discussed the use of drill as a basic therapy tool. Consistent rehearsal of the cornerstone R and the cornerstone word has been offered as a key to a successful outcome in R therapy. But drill work can be boring, a key factor in loss of motivation. We have discussed the use of stickers, stars and other rewards in R therapy, and these are quite useful. But there are other ways to help clients through the "boring" work. The following ideas are offered to help readers think about ways to make drill work tolerable, and even interesting.

MANDALLAS

A mandalla is a picture that consists of smaller pictures drawn in regular patterns around a center figure or center point. Mandallas have appeared the world over in almost all cultures. They have been used for centuries as a method of focusing the mind and as representatives of higher spiritual development. We see mandallas in the design of rugs, tapestries, clothing, stained glass, sand paintings and more. Drawing a colorful mandalla can be a nicely engaging activity for many children. It is an excellent tool for use during drill practice because children can draw one tiny piece of the drawing as a reward after each of his responses. For example, do you see the dots, lines, hearts, circles, triangles and boxes on the mandallas pictured in figure 12.1? A central element is drawn. Then the client draws one item after each of his productions. As such, the construction of the mandalla affords us an excuse for practicing the same sound or word dozens of times. Mandallas can be small and simple or large and elaborate, depending on the amount of work to be rehearsed and the intellectual development of the client. My clients usually love this process and beg to make mandallas often.

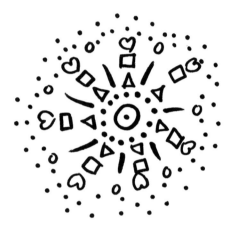

Fig. 12.1. The mandalla is a simple way to focus the mind and center it on the work of R.

CONSTRUCTION PROJECTS

Building with Leggos®, TinkerToys®, Lincoln Logs® and other construction toys is another excellent way to encourage drill on specific aspects of R therapy. The client earns, or "buys," one piece of construction equipment per utterance. Be careful with these activities, however. Many of these toys are difficult to manage in terms of the fine motor skills they require. Clients can become frustrated with them. Also, just like board games and sports activities, the construction of the object itself can draw too much of the client's attention away from the process of R therapy. Don't use these activities with clients who cannot continue to work on R while constructing, and don't let too much time be focused on the construction project itself. However, bring out the construction toys periodically to spice up a boring session that must be focused on drill.

SOMETHING TO KEEP HANDS BUSY

Recent studies have confirmed what many of us have known for years: Many children speak up more when they have something to do with their hands. Unlike the classic model of therapy that requires a client's undivided visual attention and still hands, some children—especially boys—are willing to drill on R productions and words more readily when they have something to fiddle with. Somehow engaging the hands allows them to relax and talk simultaneously. How often have parents been accused of saying, "Stop fiddling with that and listen to me!" What we are coming to see is that fiddling actually helps some children pay attention.

Once they have learned a cornerstone R, and when it does not distract from the client's production of sounds or words, I do not require any of my clients to look at me. Instead, I give them something with which to fidget, including rubberbands, paper clips, key chains, magnets or other small toys. Many of these clients will find something to fiddle with anyway, so it's best to give them permission and something interesting to use. We can always take it away when he gets off track. Then we can give it back as a reward for paying attention and doing as he is told.

DRAWING

Drawing and painting can be included in our list of ways to help clients focus. We are talking about freeform drawing, during which the client can draw whatever suits him. This can function to occupy their hands while making responses. Freeform drawings are not constructed one piece at a time like mandalla drawings. Instead, clients are allowed to draw or paint while you talk and give them sounds or words to repeat. The work is paced slowly so that a leisurely tone is set. For example, while he is drawing, the client is asked to repeat several sounds or words, and then a moment of silence follows. Then the therapist repeats a target word several times while the client listens, and a moment of silence follows. Then the client is asked to try a certain word. Praise is offered and silence follows. Every once in a while, the client is asked to put down his marker or brush, look at the therapist, and focus visual attention on her while she models a sound or word. Such integration of drawing and rehearsing can settle and engage the mind. It will not work with all clients, of course. Mature ones will do well under these conditions once they have a perfect sound to rehearse. It is a great tool for use during the later stages of therapy and for easy clients.

Assign Homework

Home practice should be a regular part of R therapy. Suggestions in the main body of our text have been made regarding what to practice at home. In this section, we summarize how to organize this practice.

PRACTICE SUCCESSFULLY

Homework is useful only when clients are practicing skills they do well. Therefore, homework should never include practicing skills not yet mastered in the therapy room. If a client is just beginning to produce a decent cornerstone R sound but is inconsistent in its production, do not encourage him to practice it at home. He probably will practice it wrong. Instead, backtrack and practice those skills he conquered just before he attained the cornerstone sound. In this way, he will get even better on his foundational skills, and the cornerstone will be even better the following week.

LIMIT TIME

It is strongly recommended that homework exercises be brief—under three minutes. Longer practices will be ignored by most clients. Make these exercises quick and easy, like they are no big deal, and make them simple. Reward the client for getting exercises done in as short a period of time as possible. If you give him an exercise that takes only one minute, praise him. "All right! You are really fast at this work!" With a little memorization, the work can be practiced any time of the day or night. A short list of three specific words will be memorized within one or two practice times. Then the words can be rehearsed dozens of times per day without referring to the notebook. It is better for our clients to practice three R words five times a day than it is to practice twenty words only once a day.

IDENTIFY LOCATIONS

Privacy is an important part of homework for 'tweens and teens. Adolescent clients do not want to be on display as they work through these oral-motor and production activities. Recommend that they practice in the bathroom in front of the mirror. Give them activities to do at the sink, in the shower, while brushing the teeth, after brushing the teeth, while combing hair, flossing teeth, and so forth. Consider assigning 30-second activities to do in bed at night, as well as silent activities to do in the car. Also, assign unobtrusive oral-motor activities to do while eating and while sitting quietly in the classroom.

LIST HOMEWORK ACTIVITIES IN THE SPEECH BINDER

Each page of the speech binder is a potential homework page and pages that are to be rehearsed at home should be marked in a special way. Ask the client how he wants you to mark the homework pages. A boy may want a green monster at the top of the pages while a girl may want a flower. Mark them according to the client's direction and he will remember which ones to do. Alternately, use the page numbering system to make a list of pages to do as homework. Special notes are written for parents to give them clues about what the child is expected to do on the homework pages if necessary. For example, write the word SLOW on pages of words the child must practice slowly.

Involve Parents

There is a joke about parent involvement I always tell in my workshops. When you work in the public schools, you think, *If I could only get the parents to come* in *here, this child's therapy would go much better.* And when you work in private practice, you think, *If I could only get the parents* out *of here, this child's therapy would go much better.*

The underlying truth is that some parents help the process of articulation therapy, while others hinder it. Some parents comply with our instructions, while others fight us over every little step all along the way. Some parents are silent, and we feel we cannot get to know them well enough to understand what they think about therapy. Other parents never stay quiet long enough for us to accomplish the day's work. Some belittle their children right in front of us. Others think their children can do no wrong. Many parents push their children too quickly into stages of therapy that are beyond the client's immediate skills. Others treat articulation therapy for their child as if it were psychological therapy for themselves.

Parent involvement in therapy needs to be discussed as part of a successful R therapy program because it can be an integral part of client motivation and success. Since parents are more consistently involved in private therapy, we shall discuss this perspective. Significant changes to these ideas will be needed for the school-based program.

We opened this chapter by saying that this material represents my personal style in R therapy. Nowhere is that more true than how it concerns working with parents. I do not recommend these procedures for any other types of speech therapy. These recommendations are for high-level R clients who are involved in individual therapy one time per week for thirty minutes only. They are not recommended for children with fluency disorder, apraxia, language disorder, and so forth. The following ideas are presented in no specific order.

TAKE CONTROL

The first step for working with the parents of R clients is to take charge of the program. Involve the parents fully in the assessment session, and then keep them out of the room for at least half of each therapy session. I begin each treatment session with the client alone. During that time, we have a little chat, review home practice, discuss problems or other issues that come up, and begin to add new practice routines. Then, once the client has acquired his personal best work of the day, I show him what exercises we are going to demonstrate to his parent. Then I ask him to go to the lobby to invite the parent in. With the parent seated at our table, the child and I continue with about three more minutes of the same work so she can observe what has been going on. This becomes a little performance. I explain the home practice, and we discuss details of schedules and so forth. I follow this routine even when I have an observation window available for parent viewing. But I do not follow it rigidly every session. Parents are not involved at all in some sessions, and sometimes I invite parents to come in and sit through an entire practice.

I have found that this routine is an excellent one for four main reasons. First, I want the client to feel that he and I are in this work alone. I want him to feel that I am in charge and that his parent is only a witness. This is so the child will depend on me and not be conflicted about whose advice he should follow in learning R. Most parents seem grateful I am in charge. They literally do not know what to do about this problem, and they want an expert to fix it. They want to wait in the lobby while the child is worked on, just like at the dentist's office. Next, parents like to see their children perform and accomplish something. They feel that they are getting their money's worth when every session includes a demonstration of the new skills. Finally, demonstrating therapy begins the process of carryover. It puts the client's new skills in front of other people right from the first day of treatment.

There are times during which parents can and will be more involved than this. Some parents insist on being in the room at all times. I allow this—at least for a little while. There usually comes a time when the parent begins to realize the child would do better alone, and they gladly retreat. Also, if a client works with me successfully when the parent is in the room, then I invite the parent in a little bit earlier each session until the entire sessions can be done with the parent present all the time.

LET PARENTS AIR FEELINGS

Parents often have years of pent-up feelings regarding their child's misarticulation of R. These need to be aired, especially when the parents have adopted a negative attitude about their child's misarticulation. Remember, many clients have been in years of prior R therapy with little or no success. Hopelessness may have set in regarding a child's lack of progress. Or the parent may believe their child is simply not trying hard enough. Parents may blame themselves for not bringing the child to therapy early enough, or may express guilt they have not been able to help the child themselves. They may be mad that the child does not qualify for school therapy. And there may be issues regarding the child's willingness to participate that the parent is unable to address.

Therapists must be sensitive to the subtle signs that reveal these issues and must be willing to discuss them openly. Children may have to leave the room if parents feel uncomfortable talking about their fears and their frustrations when the children are present. Ask the child to leave, and do not reveal to him what you and the parent are discussing. This is a private matter, just as is the work he is doing with you. Also use private time with the parents to talk about the child and his reaction to therapy.

ADJUST PARENT'S EXPECTATIONS

One of the most important things we do with parents is to help stabilize their expectations of success. This can mean bringing expectations down or lifting them up. Some parents feel such hopelessness, and they need help to see how well their child is doing in the process of learning R. These parents need help learning to celebrate the small steps. Other parents have such high expectations of their child that they expect him to fly through the program. They may insist that their child try things over his head. These parents have to learn how to stay quiet about skills they think their child should already be able to do. They need to back off, learn patience, and wait through the necessary small steps.

CONTROL NEGATIVE COMMENTS

Some clients have family members, either parents or siblings, who tease or belittle them because of their misarticulated R. These things need to be discussed with the family. Those comments need to be curbed. Many parents need help understanding that their comments have a huge impact on their child's willingness to work on R. Family members need to see the production of correct R as a skill to be learned, not as a character flaw in their child.

TRAIN PARENTS TO HEAR R

Most parents cannot hear a correct R when it finally emerges in their child. I watch parents carefully as the child and I demonstrate skills. Once a child begins to produce a correct cornerstone R sound, many parents must strain to hear it. They try to recognize the correctness of the sound, but the look on their faces tells me they cannot. The child's utterance does not sound like the R they were expecting. They struggle to understand why I am enthusiastic about the funny sound I assure them is a good one. This is the time to bring parents in therapy a little more each session. It will train them to hear the sound. If parents are the key people at home to monitor practice activities, they need to be able to tell when R is correct and when it is not. Parents are not at fault for this lack of skill. They simply are not yet trained to hear R at a therapy level.

HELP PARENTS SEE THE BIG PICTURE

One of the most difficult tasks in R therapy is to inform parents that their particular child has a bigger problem than a simple misarticulation of R. I am always amazed when parents call me to set up an evaluation and tell me that the child has trouble with R but has no other problem. Then the client arrives and I see problems with attention, language processing, oral-motor skills, dysarthria and so forth. I usually say, "I hear the problem with R, but it seems that there are more problems. Do you ever have trouble understanding him?" This usually helps the parent begin to talk about the whole picture and not just the problem with R. I take this opportunity to inform the parents that these other characteristics are probably the reason the child has had trouble. I tell them R is "the hardest sound in the world." When kids have other subtle speech problems, R can be delayed in emergence. This helps parents understand why we will be working on other speech skills as well as R. It also helps them see why therapy will take more than just a few weeks.

RELIEVE SLPS OF THEIR GUILT

Speech and language pathologists with children who haven't learned R usually carry tremendous guilt. Imagine what it would feel like to have a child who cannot do the very thing you are supposed to be able to fix. These SLPs need to understand three things. First, they need to realize that not every therapist is an expert on R, and they shouldn't worry so much about it. Point out therapy lapses in your own treatment experiences. I tell other therapists that I have little real experience when it comes to fluency therapy. I explain that if one of my children stuttered, I would be heading straight for another expert. Parents need to realize you don't think any less of them because they have not been able to change their own child's R.

Second, SLPs need to realize that being the parent of a child who cannot say R is quite different from being his therapist. Children will do things for therapists they would never do for parents. These therapists need to realize they have a different relationship with their child, and they need to see that it is more important for them to maintain their role as the child's parent than it is for them to take on the role of his therapist. The child does not need role confusion in his life. It is better that the parent not introduce it. These therapists need reassurance that it is okay not to be their own child's therapist.

Third, SLPs need to be told that their child's performance in therapy and the personal things you discuss about their family in the process are confidential, just like it would be for any other client. This policy may be assumed, but I find it important to state this fact outright. It helps everyone relax.

Summary

- Motivating participation draws clients into the process of learning R. It makes them want to say perfect R's all the time, and it ensures carryover. Motivation is one of the most challenging aspects of R therapy.

- Chronological age is a significant factor in designing an R therapy program that captures a client's attention. In general, the younger the client, the more the therapy will look like play. The older the client, the more the therapy will look like academic work.

- Chronological age also determines the emotional demands of the program. Younger children can be tricked into producing a correct R. Older 'tweens and teens will have to make their own decision to change their R sound.

- Successful R therapy includes discussion about the unique nature of R. Many clients need to understand that R is a rare and difficult sound, and that it takes a long time to learn it.

- Clients who engage in the difficult work of R therapy should be rewarded for their efforts. The purpose of a reward system is to get the client on track and to keep him there through the long haul of R therapy. Rewards need to be meaningful to the client. The ultimate reward of R therapy should be the acquisition of R itself.

- Clients and their parents need to know how long R therapy will take. Clients often accept a treatment program if they know when they can get out. It is recommended that R therapy be scheduled for short definitive periods of time that can be repeated.

- Each session of treatment should add tiny new elements to what already has been accomplished. Tiny steps ensure that clients practice only that which they can do very well. This solidifies skills and creates the impression that the work is easy.

- An old-fashioned speech binder can be a permanent record of all the work a client does in therapy. It is constructed page by page by the therapist and client. It is a wonderful way to review material and keep parents informed about treatment. A binder is an amazing way for a client to track his progress and a great way for multiple therapists to keep track of each other's treatment goals and activities.

- Children of elementary age and older who are enrolled in R therapy should be stimulated to think about why they come to therapy. A mind that is engaged in the process will create faster and more solid changes. A focused mind helps a client become more deeply committed to the process of change and it ensures better carryover.

- Therapists must take a good look at their therapy programs to determine if too much time is wasted on games and other activities. Activities should not detract a client from learning the R sound.

- Drill is a basic therapy tool for automating the production of a correct R. Drill work can be made tolerable and even interesting with drawings and construction projects.

- Homework is useful only when clients are practicing skills they do well in the therapy room. Make homework exercises quick and easy. It is better to practice for one minute every day than to practice for twenty minutes one time per week.

- Parent involvement contributes to a successful R program. It is integral to client motivation and success. Parents usually like therapists to take charge of the program. We should help parents air their feelings, adjust their expectations, control their negative comments, see the big picture and hear their child's new correct R.

- Parents who are also speech and language pathologists present special cases. We should encourage them to maintain their role of parent and relinquish their role as therapist. We should assure them that it is natural for their children to work better with another adult.

#13 Assuring Persistent Success
Final Words of Advice on Successful R Therapy

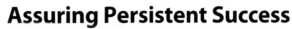

I have been trying to write this book for nearly twenty years. It has always been a part of me, but I could not put it on paper until now. I needed more years of experimentation with R before I would be able to write sufficiently to help other speech and language pathologists. It takes a long time to feel comfortable with and truly successful in changing the wide variety of errors seen in R therapy. Some R's practically fix themselves; others are as stubborn as mules.

Here is a summary of advice for reaching persistent success in R therapy. These ideas are presented in no particular order. I hope they help you, and the profession at large, improve success in R therapy.

- *Difficulty:* Don't panic if the client is getting nowhere. R therapy can be very difficult with some clients. When stuck, get a new perspective on how your client is misarticulating his sound. Sit back, watch his mouth carefully and listen closely. Consider watching the client speak while you both look into a mirror. The reverse image can give a new perspective. And there may be more fundamental problems with his speech. Shift your focus to some of these to shore up his foundational skills.
- *Junk:* Do not accept bad productions, or *junk*. Train your ear to hear a good R. Don't be sloppy in your range of acceptable phonemes. Look for one perfect R and accept no substitutes!
- *Expression:* Allow yourself to express great joy when a client achieves his early R sounds. Celebrate! Praise him! Tell him how awesome he is. Show off his skill to others. Help him realize that you are on his side, you like him and you honor his hard work. Let him know you will march with him through his own battle with R.
- *Time:* Give yourself time to perfect the skill of R therapy. Years. However long it takes you, that's how long it takes. Do your best with every client. Use each client to teach you more about the way to successful R productions.
- *Bravery:* Try new things. Don't get stuck in a rut doing the same methods year after year, especially if they are not working. Try something new—anything. Shake

things up. Take your clients off the familiar track and give them a big shove onto a new one.
- *Creativity:* Design methods that make sense for you, and figure out why they work. Try new techniques and figure out how to modify them to fit the client's need.
- *Observation:* Watch other therapists do R therapy. Even if she is the worst therapist in the world, you will learn from her. Her bunglings will help shape your therapy. Of course, you may be watching the best speech and language pathologist in the world. In that case, watch very carefully, and absorb her techniques and her demeanor.
- *Conferences:* One generally doesn't see much in the way of R Therapy conferences, but if you find one, go! Especially if it will have a practical focus. Be sure to attend if the speaker is a frontline speech and language pathologist with many years on the job in articulation therapy.
- *Take and Give:* Take in every new idea from other therapists, and give them what you know about R therapy. Every technique is valuable, no matter its genre and source. Host an informal successful-R party with a small group of like-minded therapists as a place to give advice freely to one another. Make your motto: "All techniques have value!" Share this book and other materials on R therapy.
- *Lend a Hand:* Give a guest lecture on R therapy to university students ready to enter the workforce. These poor kids probably know nothing about the phoneme they are about to face the next year. A new crop of speech and language pathologists emerges from the universities every year, so make it your annual mission to help the new generation of students face R with some skill. Be very practical in the talk. Use the exercises offered in this book as small group activities to be done in the workshop. Help new therapists understand oral-motor patterns involved in R production and misarticulation, and to recognize the value of auditory training in the remediation process.
- *Oral-Motor Therapy:* Don't believe the naysayers who claim that oral-motor therapy has no effect on articulation improvement. They don't know what they are talking about. Speech is movement. Period. One cannot change articulation precision without making changes to oral movement. How could one bring changes to a distorted R if one were to leave oral movements unchanged? Even the earliest of our clinician/researcher/scholar/writers knew this. People like Sara Stinchfield Hawk, Charles Van Riper, Lee Edward Travis, and Frederick Darley wrote frequently about oral-motor therapy, although they did not use that term. Oral-motor therapy simply brings organization and science to mouth exercises.
- *Clients:* Let the clients show you what they are interested in and what they want to do in therapy. Your therapy will improve. But don't let them take over. Then your therapy will deteriorate.
- *Parents:* Don't be intimidated by parents. You don't have to answer their every need. Let parents know what *you* need. Let them watch from the sidelines. Don't assume that parents know anything about articulation therapy or behavior management. Don't let them derail you. Include parents in therapy when they are a benefit to it, but keep them out if they detract from the process.

- *Referrals:* Refer to an R specialist in private practice, if possible. Some clients simply need it.
- *Specializing:* Become a specialist in R therapy yourself. Private practice needs people who really understand how to fix R sounds. And, just like every school district needs an augmentative communication specialist, every district also needs an R pro to help with difficult cases.
- *Failed Techniques:* Don't abandon techniques just because they don't work with the first client or with the first ten clients. Keep them around for the right client who is coming down the pike.
- *Time Off:* Don't be afraid to postpone or take a break from treatment. Re-enroll the client later when there is a better chance of success. General maturity plays a big role in the learning process. But don't miss a prime opportunity to help a younger child who is ready. Use professional judgment.
- *Review:* Reread this book in a year or so. Techniques that made no sense the first time will come to light after you see more clients. Then read it again in another few years.
- *Published Materials:* Published R therapy workbooks, cards and games are a good source of material that can contribute mightily to a successful R therapy program. But don't use only published material. Pre-printed lists and workbook pages will not address R with the kind of detail we have described here.
- *Prevention:* Teach preschool, kindergarten and first-grade teachers the basics of R production to use while they are teaching R in their phonics lessons. Teach both the Tip R and the Back R. Help them discover their own habitual position. Pique their interest in this phoneme so they become interested in how they and their own students produce the sounds. Consider presenting this in a short inservice meeting. These teachers may be able to help the easiest kids avoid R therapy, and they will be better at spotting the ones who need direct treatment.
- *Quiet Environments:* Insist that your articulation work take place outside of the regular classroom. Don't let the politically correct "working in the classroom" language model change what you know about articulation therapy. It is better to retreat to a quiet broomcloset than work in a noisy classroom. If challenged, ask, "Where should your child take piano lessons? In the middle of a busy classroom or in an intimate and quiet environment?" They'll get the picture.
- *Fun:* Have fun! Articulation therapy can be one of the most satisfying experiences. No joke. Leading a bright child from a terrible distortion of R to a truly beautiful acoustic *ring!* as he pronounces R in his everyday conversational speech is nothing short of a small miracle. I see speech therapy as a process of using one's gifts as a teacher and facilitator to help people attain the gift of good speech. This process should not be drudgery. Sessions that drag usually take clients nowhere. Sessions that are interesting and intriguing, however, capture our clients' imaginations and make them feel like they are having fun. Lead them to higher ground by laughing more and moaning less.

- *Devotion:* The great number of R words that appear as practice in this text should help readers realize how important R is to the English language. How can a person be understood well and respected if he mispronounces a phoneme that is so important to the language? The staggering number of R sounds most people utter per day reveals just how important our work is. Speech and language pathologists should be devoted to R's correct production. We should not let go of this important work.

Each small skill learned along the way is a significant step upward on the path of successful R therapy. Create an atmosphere of mounting success as you work toward the day when your client will have learned everything possible about producing R correctly. Savor the pleasure of each stage, and allow yourself to experience the pure joy of dismissing a client from a successful program. Know in your heart that you are doing good things for people who are struggling in a small yet extremely important part of their lives. There is a joy and pride one feels when one hears excellent R's in former clients who are now teachers, doctors, politicians, construction workers, bankers, mothers and fathers. This is the dignity of our work. The success that comes to people's lives after we help them learn to pronounce R makes all the struggles of this therapy worth the effort.

Glossary

acoustic flavor. The characteristic sound quality of a particular phoneme.

apex. Target position of speech movement in phoneme production. It occurs between the on-glide and the off-glide movements. The apex of R is where the ultimate position of the sound is achieved and isolated R is heard.

apraxia. a non-linguistic sensorimotor disorder of articulation characterized by decreased capacity to program the movements of speech.

articulation. The way phonemes are formed in the throat and mouth.

auditory bombardment. The presentation of multiple examples of target sounds in words spoken by the therapist to a client who is engaged in a quiet activity.

auditory stimulus. A specific auditory event provided for auditory training. Auditory stimuli are used to help clients hear R as a distinct unit of sound and to discriminate fine differences in its production.

babbling. The process of rehearsing sequences of consonants and vowels that emerge in infants by six or seven months of age. Babbling in infancy is done for pleasure, self-entertainment and sound discovery, rather than general communication purposes.

baby talk. The common and expected speech patterns of young children.

backing. In phonological terms, the process of substituting sounds made in the back of the oral mechanism for those made in the front (k/t, g/d, ŋ/n, r/l, etc.).

beat. The periodic production of throbs or pulsations in speech.

carryover. A traditional term for the process of using the speech skills one has learned in therapy to speaking situations outside of the therapy room, with other conversational partners, and under other speaking conditions.

classic back R distortion. Common distortion of R caused as a client attempts a Back R. Specifically, instead of lifting and stabilizing the back-lateral margins of the tongue, the client lifts and tenses the middle back while leaving the back margins low and lax.

co-articulation. The influence of movement from one speech sound to another within a sequence formed by a word or across words.

consonant. Voiced or voiceless speech sound made with constriction, namely /p/, /b/, /t/, /d/, /k/, /g/, /m/, /n/, /ŋ/, /w/, /l/, /y/, /r/, /f/, /v/, /θ/, /ð/, /s/, /z/, /ʃ/, /ʒ/, /tʃ/, /dʒ/, /h/.

consonantal R. The sound of R as it occurs at the beginning of a syllable and before a vowel. The Consonantal R is written with only one IPA symbol: /r/.

conversational games. Verbal games that incorporate a cornerstone word.

cornerstone sound. The first correct R sound a client can produce consistently over trials.

cornerstone word. A single word that perfectly reflects a client's cornerstone sound.

Demosthenes. An orator from Athens, Greece, who died in 322 B.C. Demosthenes reportedly spoke with marbles in his mouth in order to learn to enunciate clearly. Widely regarded as the first known speech student.

developmental error. A speech sound error that is expected to occur in normal development.

dialogue. Discourse between two speakers.

diphthong. A sound comprised of two distinct vowel resonances and the sound made while transitioning from the first to the second.

distortion. Mispronunciation of speech sounds caused by imprecise speech movement. The inaccurate twisting or bending of speech sounds.

duration of voice. Length of time during which sound (voice) is produced.

dysarthria. A motor-speech disorder affecting respiration, phonation, resonation and articulation. Dysarthria causes distortion of speech sound.

dysarthric. Having the characteristics of dysarthria.

facilitate. To cause (a movement) to occur.

finely graded open position. The optimal position of jaw during production of speech. A slightly lowered position of the jaw so that the mouth is held somewhat open.

frenectomy. In surgery, the removal of a frenum. The lingual frenectomy releases the tension of the short or restricting lingual frenum. The term *z-plasty* is used and refers to a z-shaped incision made in the frenum.

frenum. Fold of skin or mucous membrane that limits the movement of an organ. The lingual frenum is a small, white cord of tissue extending from the floor of the mouth to the middle of the inferior surface of the tongue. When too short, the lingual frenum can restrict upward elevation and lateral extension of the tongue tip.

glide. Speech sounds made during articulatory movement, specifically W, L, Y and R.

hypernasality. Too much nasality produced in speech; sound traveling through the nasal passageways when it shouldn't.

idiosyncrasy. A habit or mannerism that is peculiar to an individual.

idiosyncratic distortion. A distortion of a sound that is unique to an individual client.

idiosyncratic hierarchy of R therapy. A therapy program designed for one client and built around his cornerstone sound.

Individualized Educational Plan (IEP). A written treatment plan that includes goals, objectives, procedures, success criteria and outcomes. The IEP is signed by the speech and language pathologist and parents or other guardians. Other school personnel may be included. The speech and language IEP is updated on a regular basis.

inhibit. To prevent (a movement) from occurring.

intelligibility. The degree to which a client can be understood. A client who is 100 percent intelligible can be understood virtually all the time. At 50 percent, a client can be understood about half the time, and so forth.

intensity. Energy, strength or magnitude of voice.

intonation. The pattern of pitch changes in connected speech.

intrusive R. An R that creeps in where it does not belong.

isolated R. The sound of true R as heard when the tongue is at its apex of movement. The isolated R is made by on-gliding and off-gliding in silence. Voice is produced only when the tongue is at its highest point.

labial. Pertaining to the lips.

labialization. The substitute of a labial (lip) sound for a lingual (tongue) sound.

labio-dental. Referring to the lips (labio) and the teeth (denta). Labio-dental phonemes in English include /f/ and /v/.

lingual. Pertaining to the tongue.

lingual frenum (lingua frenum). A small, white cord of tissue extending from the floor of the mouth to the middle of the inferior surface of the tongue. When too short, the lingual frenum can restrict upward elevation of the tongue tip. (See also *frenum* and *frenectomy*.)

lip retractor. A device designed to pull the lips laterally. When placed on the lips, it helps the tongue to move differentially from the lips.

lisp. A defective production of one or more of the six sibilant sounds. Patterns include dental, frontal, interdental, nasal, occluded and lateral lisps.

Melodic Intonation Therapy. A program of speech therapy that utilizes specific regular intonation patterns to aid in speech sound production and sequencing.

minimal pairs. Pairs of words alike in all sounds except one—e.g., *bus/but*, *car/jar*, and *hat/hit*.

monologue. a prolonged talk by a single speaker.

morpheme. The smallest unit of speech with meaning—e.g., *-ing*.

negative practice. The purposeful incorrect practice of a target phoneme in order to experience, understand and take control if its production.

neutral position of the tongue. The posture assumed by the tongue when it is at rest. Also called the *resting posture*. In neutral, the tongue lies low in the oral cavity. It fits neatly inside the arch of the upper and lower dental arches. The upper surface of the tongue tip tends to articulate with the alveolar ridge, the sides tend to rest gently against the sides of the palate, and the middle and back tend to rest low and away from the palate.

normal range. The extent of variations that are all considered as acceptable and correct.

off-glide. Movement away from a phoneme's target position. The final movements of a phoneme's production.

omission. The absence of a phoneme.

on-glide. Movement toward a phoneme's target position. The first movements of a phoneme.

onset of voice. The initiation of sound in phoneme production.

oral habits. Acquired behavior patterns involving the mouth.

oral stereognosis. The process of identifying type and location of objects in the mouth through the sense of touch; oral form recognition.

oral-motor. Referring to mouth movement, specifically jaw, lip and tongue movement.

oral-motor therapy. The process of facilitating improved oral (jaw, lip, tongue) movement.

oration. Formal speech, especially speech delivered in front of a group.

orofacial myofunctional therapist. A professional with particular expertise in eliminating reverse or infantile swallowing patterns, in facilitating appropriate oral-rest position, and in eliminating oral habits.

over-articulate. To pronounce with exaggeration yet without distortion.

phoneme. "A linguistic unit consisting of a group, or family, of sounds that are not identical but that may be used interchangeably within words without affecting their meaning" (Carrell and Tiffany, 1960, p. 19).

phonetics. The study of speech sounds.

phonology. The study of the sound system of a language and the rules governing their organization into syllables.

pitch. The amplitude and frequency of sound.

placeholder. A developmentally less mature phoneme used in place of a later developing phoneme.

position sense of a phoneme. Sensations arising from the muscles and joints involved as a phoneme is produced; proprioception.

proprioception. Sensation arising from muscles and joints.

proprioceptive stimuli. Input provided to the muscles and joints in order to facilitate an adaptive response (movement).

prosody. Attributes of speech that signal linguistic function—i.e., stress and intonation, melody of speech.

protrude. To thrust forward, anteriorly, to the forward part of the mouth.

quality of voice. Timbre of sound produced at the vocal folds.

R quality. The acoustic signal that marks the sound of R.

range of acceptability. The limits within which a phoneme can vary and still be considered correct.

rapport. The harmonious or sympathetic relationship between client and therapist.

rate. Degree of speed at which phonemes, syllables and words are produced within an utterance.

resonance. Sympathetic vibration of air and sound in the mouth, nose and other facial cavities.

resting posture of the tongue. (See *neutral position of the tongue.*)

retract. To pull back, toward the back of the mouth or head.

rhythm of speech. Uniform or patterned recurrence of beat in syllable and word.

root word. A basic word or stem from which other words are derived

schwa. A neutral vowel; a vowel made with the mouth slightly open while the tongue remains in neutral position.

self-correction. The ability to notice one's own speech-sound errors and to make an immediate correction without being prompted.

signature distortion. A distortion of a phoneme that is peculiar to an individual.

speed limits in speech production. A client's understanding of rate of speech and its relationship to accuracy of sound production. Clients must understand how to speed up and slow down their own utterances in order to produce good R sounds under various speech conditions.

stimulation techniques. Methods capable of eliciting a response.

stimulability. The degree to which a client responds to treatment techniques.

strength of voice. Power in sound production.

stress. Patterns of relative loudness and quietness used on syllables in words

substitution. A replacement of one phoneme for another.

successive approximations. A phoneme-shaping tool based on the systematic reward of phoneme productions that are increasingly closer to the target sound.

super-articulate. To pronounce in a big way without distortion.

synchronistic productions. Two identical speech sounds made at the same time by two people.

systematic babbling. A rhythmic approach to sequential phoneme practice with R and other phonemes; an organized babbling repertoire.

tactics. Procedures that guide the overall process of articulation treatment.

tactile stimuli. Input provided to the cutaneous tissue (skin) in order to emit an adaptive response (movement).

target position. The pinnacle of speech movement where the ultimate position of the sound is achieved and direction of movement changes. A phoneme's target position occurs between its on-glide and its off-glide.

TBR. (See *Tongue Bowl Response.*)

techniques. Auditory, visual and oral-motor procedures designed to bring about the correct acoustic quality of the R sound.

termination of voice. The end point of sound production in phoneme pronunciation.

Tongue Bowl Response. The cup or bowl-shaped configuration assumed by the tongue in response to tactile stimulation provided down the midline of the tongue from tip to back. The tongue should flatten, flair out from midline, elevate its perimeter and depress its middle in response to such stimuli.

traditional articulation therapy. Speech correction plans and procedures proposed by the earliest researchers in the field of speech and language therapy. Techniques in popular use before the introduction of phonological and oral-motor techniques.

transitioning. Moving into and out of a phoneme's apex position.

treasure chest. A container of small objects to be used as rewards for good participation or performance in therapy.

vibrotactile sensations. Tactile sensations that result from sound vibration.

visual stimuli. Cues that can be seen. Visual stimuli are used to help clients understand how the jaw, lips and tongue move in and out of position for production of a sound.

vocal play. Playful experimentation with vocal sound productions.

vocalic. Made with voice.

vocalic R. The sound of R as it occurs at the end of a syllable after a vowel. The Vocalic R is written with several different IPA symbols, depending upon the preceding vowel.

voice. Sound produced by the vocal folds.

vowel. A voiced speech sound made without restriction on the air stream. Standard English orthography employs six vowels, namely A, E, I, O, U and Y. The International Phonetic Alphabet includes many more for the English language, including /i/, /ɪ/, /e/, /ɛ/, /æ/, /u/, /ʊ/, /o/, /ɔ/, /ɑ/, /ʌ/ and /ə/.

References

Carrell, James and William Tiffany, (1960). *Phonetics: Theory and Application to Speech Improvement.* McGraw-Hill Book Company: New York, New York.

Hanson, Marvin, (1983). *Articulation.* W. B. Saunders Company: Philadelphia, Pennsylvania.

Hodson, Barabara Williams and Elaine Pagel Paden, (1983). *Targeting Intelligible Speech.* College-Hill Press: San Diego, California.

Marshalla, Pam, (2001). *How to Stop Drooling.* Marshalla Speech and Language: Kirkland, Washington.

Marshalla, Pam, (2001). *How to Stop Thumbsucking.* Marshalla Speech and Language: Kirkland, Washington.

Marshalla, Pam, (2001). *Oral-Motor Techniques in Articulation and Phonological Therapy.* Marshalla Speech and Language: Kirkland, Washington.

Nicolosi, Lucille, Elizabeth Harryman and Janet Kresheck, (1983). *Terminology of Communication Disorders.* Williams and Wilkins: Baltimore, Maryland.

Zemlin, Willard (1968). *Speech and Hearing Science.* Prentice-Hall, Inc.: Englewood Cliffs, New Jersey.

Appendix A
Functional Zones of the Tongue

Although the tongue is considered one single body part, its musculature allows it to move various areas differentially for the production of speech sounds. Analysis of palatography data has revealed 16 independent moving parts or *functional zones* of the tongue. Based on this data, new assignments of tongue areas have been given. The schematic illustration below specifies these parts. Please see *Oral-motor Techniques in Articulation and Phonological Therapy* for more on this.

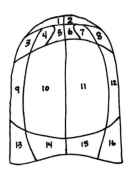

Fig. A.1. Functional Zones of the Tongue

Tip: zones 1, 2
Blade: zones 4, 5, 6, 7
Lateral Blade: zones 4, 7
Middle Blade: zones 5, 6
Body: zones 10, 11
Back: zones 13, 14, 15, 16
Lateral Backs: zones 13, 16
Middle Back: zones 14, 15
Left Lateral Margin: zones 3, 9, 13
Right Lateral Margin: zones 8, 12, 16

Appendix B
Sample Evaluation Report

Name: Robert Everybody
Date of Evaluation: 07-24-2003
Birthdate: 05-19-1990
Age at Evaluation: 13 years, 2 months
Parents: Mr. and Mrs. Everybody
Address: 12345 Any Street
   Anytown, USA
Telephone: 555-555-5555

Background
Robert was referred by his school speech and language pathologist, Sarah Speaker. The concern was need for extra help in pronunciation of R because he has received two years of speech therapy for R with little improvement. Development in all other areas seems to be within normal limits. Robert has had no other speech, language or learning problems in school. He had a few ear infections as a young child, but these subsided with antibiotics and he has passed several hearing screenings at school and at his pediatrician's office. Robert sucked his thumb until six years of age and currently wears braces. Orthodontics is under the direction of Dr. Braces of Anytown USA.

Examination
No formal evaluation tools were used today. Instead, direct observation of spontaneous and imitated speech, response to selected treatment techniques, and discussion with the client and his mother comprised our main forms of assessment.

Speech
Robert demonstrated a distortion of R in all contexts of words. He was unable to produce a correct R today despite many treatment trials. Robert is difficult to understand in rapid conversational speech due to mispronunciation of R and some adjacent vowels. Both L and N are slightly distorted by interdental tongue placement intermittently. He has been attempting a Back R.

Oral Movement
Direct observation of the oral mechanism revealed an anterior open bite and corrective braces. No other structural deviations were noted. Tongue movements were incompletely differentiated from jaw movements, and the jaw was unstable in speech. Robert had difficulty elevating and curling the tip of the tongue. When asked how he was trying to make a correct R, Robert said he was "lifting the back." When asked to demonstrate, he retracted the entire tongue into the oropharynx.

Auditory Discrimination
Robert easily differentiated correct and incorrect R sounds produced by the therapist today, and he is highly aware that his R sound is incorrect. He and his mother were unaware, however, that the vowels and other consonants were affected.

Motivation
Robert is highly motivated to change his R sound at this time. He stated, "I hate it when people can't understand me." He is especially concerned about pronouncing his name correctly when he enters high school next year.

Summary and Recommendations
Robert demonstrates incorrect production of R in all contexts. It is recommended that weekly therapy be initiated. Both the Back R and the Tip R should be explored. Oral-motor therapy will need to be included to facilitate improved jaw and tongue control for R. The R phoneme should be taught within the broader context of correct pronunciation of the vowels and other glides and nasals.

It has been a pleasure to work with Robert and his mother today. I look forward to continued association with them.

Theresa Talker, MA, CCC-SLP
Speech and Language Pathologist

Appendix C
Sample Letter to a Physician Regarding a Restricting Lingua Frenum

Dear Dr. Medicine:

I am writing in regard to a restricting lingua frenum in our mutual patient, Ronnie Roderick. Ronnie was referred to me for speech assessment on 02-19-03. He has a minor speech problem on R and other phonemes that have not remediated despite two years of speech therapy at school. I believe that the restricting lingua frenum is the cause of his limited progress. The moderate degree to which Ronnie's lingua frenum is restricted has ramifications for several areas:

- Speech: Ronnie is unable to completely elevate the tip of the tongue away from the floor of the mouth. This causes mispronunciation many sounds, namely: T, D, N, L, S, and Z. Although a restricted lingua frenum will not prevent the emergence of R, per se, it has an overall detrimental effect on the development of the tongue movements necessary for mature speech. Freeing the tip will allow correct speech to develop.
- Eating: Without the ability to elevate the tongue tip, Ronnie has settled on an infantile suckle-swallowing pattern that he uses in all eating tasks. This also has been called a "reverse swallow pattern" or a "tongue thrust." Ronnie is unable to use correct tongue movements for side-to-side food transfer, and he cannot adequately form a bolus for swallowing. Ronnie avoids many foods because of this problem.
- Teeth: The habitual suckle-swallow pattern seems to be putting enormous pressure on the front teeth and appears to be related to the anterior open bite. The lingua restrictions also prevent him from using the tongue tip to remove food particles from the teeth between brushings. Orthodontia is pending according to the mother.
- Appearance: The restricting lingua frenum has negative social implications dues to the different appearance of tongue and jaw movements. Ronnie is concerned about what other kids think of him because of his "funny tongue."

I am asking that you refer Ronnie for oral surgery to release the tongue tip. I have talked to the mother about the reason for this referral and have suggested that she follow through with this recommendation.

Thank You,

Theresa Talker, MA, CCC-SLP
Speech and Language Pathologist

Postscript

The final draft of this book took about three years to write. I worked on it in bits and pieces during the years when my three daughters were enrolled in junior high and high school. One day I discovered that my fifteen-year-old had typed a secret note at the very end of the draft. Apparently she wanted to see how long it would take me to discover it. Now if you have raised teenagers, you know how rare certain statements become during that period, so please indulge me as I leave this note just as it appeared at the end of my unfinished document:

"HI MOM! I LUV U!!"

More by Pam Marshalla

Apraxia Uncovered — 3 audio CDs & 166-page book $89.95
The Seven Stages of Phoneme Development
A revolutionary audio seminar in articulation, phonological, and oral-motor therapy. Discover the seven stages of sound acquisition and apply it immediately to your therapy. This innovative program integrates proven essentials from articulation, phonology, oral-motor, and infant vocal development into a comprehensive program of treatment for all consonants and vowels. Nearly 30 years of clinical research together with Pam's famous practical style!

How to Stop Thumbsucking $14.95
How to Stop Drooling $14.95
Pam Marshalla's How-to Series gives you easy-to-understand resources that help to reduce or eliminate your child's thumbsucking and excessive drooling. Includes practical guidelines, solutions, and activities for home or therapy.

Becoming Verbal with Childhood Apraxia $19.95
New Insights on Piaget for Today's Therapy
Particularly relevant for minimally verbal children who have been diagnosed with apraxia or dyspraxia of speech. Includes the organization and facilitation of early sound and word emergence.

Oral Motor Techniques in Articulation and Phonological Therapy $49.95
Includes all the basics of oral-motor therapy for improving jaw, lip, and tongue control, and for normalizing oral-tactile sensitivity. Written for both the professional and student speech-language pathologist, the text guides the reader through fundamental techniques used in treatment. An excellent supplemental text for courses on motor speech disorders, articulation, phonology, feeding, and dysphagia.

Successful R Therapy $49.95
Learn how to train the most difficult R clients. From the cornerstone R to conversational speech, this takes you through every stage of articulation therapy for the misarticulated R. Includes deep insights into the relationships between oral-motor skills, auditory processing and articulation control.

Order Today

1 Select titles

Title	Price	Quantity	Total
How to Stop Thumbsucking	$14.95		$
How to Stop Drooling	$14.95		$
Becoming Verbal with Developmental Apraxia	$19.95		$
Oral-Motor Techniques	$49.95		$
Successful R Therapy	$49.95		$
Apraxia Uncovered	$89.95		$
Wholesale prices available on request			
SHIPPING AND HANDLING (1–4 books = $3.95; 5–10 books = $7.50)			$
WA residents add 8.9% sales tax			$
		TOTAL	$

2 Find total

3 Mail order

Send check or money order to
Marshalla Speech and Language
11417 - 124th Ave NE, #202
Kirkland, WA 98033

Questions?
(425) 828-4361
www.pammarshalla.com

Name:
Street:
City:
State:_____ Zip: _____
Phone: (____)
E-mail:

MSL
Marshalla Speech and Language

www.PamMarshalla.com